Nursing Rituals, Research and Rational Actions

Mike Walsh BA, RGN, PGCE, DipN
Senior Lecturer, Department of Nursing Studies, Bristol Polytechnic

and

Pauline Ford RGN, CMS
Professional Adviser in the Care of Elderly People, Royal College of Nursing, London

Foreword by Trevor Clay MPhil, RGN, RMN, FRCN
General Secretary, Royal College of Nursing 1982–1989

Cartoons by Kipper Williams

Heinemann Nursing

Heinemann Nursing
An imprint of Heinemann Professional Publishing Ltd
Halley Court, Jordan Hill, Oxford OX2 8EJ
OXFORD LONDON SINGAPORE
NAIROBI IBADAN KINGSTON

First published 1989
Reprinted 1990 (twice)

British Library Cataloguing in Publication Data

Walsh, Mike
Nursing.
1. Medicine. Nursing
I. Title   II. Ford, Pauline
610.73

ISBN 0 433 00080 5

Typeset by Lasertext Ltd, Stretford, Manchester M32 0JT
Printed and bound in Great Britain by
Biddles Ltd, Guildford and King's Lynn

NURSING RITUALS,
RESEARCH AND RATIONAL ACTIONS

Contents

Foreword

I am very pleased indeed to welcome this book which makes a significant contribution to a much neglected area of nursing. The writers make early mention of the work of Isabel Menzies and others who have looked at the whole business of rituals and ritualistic behaviour in nursing. A major debate within the profession regarding the effect nursing work has on its practitioners is long overdue. We assume that men and women who enter nursing are a different kind of human being and that they automatically possess the gifts, talents and abilities to cope with everything the profession demands of them. It is a fact of course that they cope in different ways, sometimes at great cost to themselves and sometimes at a cost to their patients. We have not yet emerged from the era where nursing treatment and care routines are not wholly geared towards the needs of patients and clients but are geared towards the providers of care or the institutions where it is provided. Mike Walsh and Pauline Ford have chosen bravely to look in detail at the behaviour of nurses and the impact it has on the nursing care and treatment they provide. They have concentrated on the rituals both of practice and of the organization. Their book is written in a way which makes it understandable by practising nurses at all levels. It is easy to read and positive in that it makes recommendations for good practice at the end of each section. I very much hope that it will be used as a tool for peer group review, for teaching — both formal and informal — and that it will be the subject of argument and debate in these forums. The book lifts the eyes of the nursing profession away from its navel and is another sign that the profession is addressing the whole area of the quality of its practice and the care of its practitioners.

Trevor Clay MPhil, RGN, RMN, FRCN
General Secretary, Royal College of Nursing 1982–1989

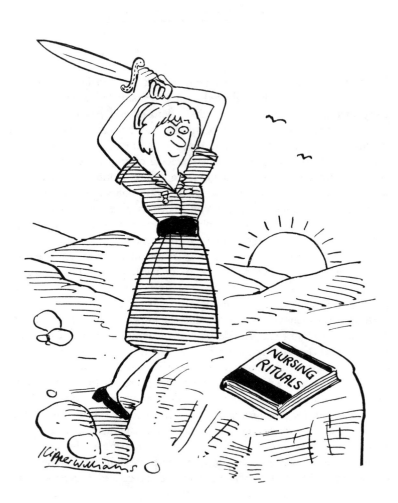

Introduction

The nurse is and remains primarily the agent of the older person, not of the institution for which he or she works (RCN Association for Care of the Elderly, 1988).

These words were originally written about the care of the elderly, but can clearly be extended to include all patients, regardless of age. The theme of the nurse being accountable to the patient, rather than to institutions and establishments, forms the basis of this book.

The reader will be familiar with books that tell you how to do things, such as how to nurse elderly people or patients requiring surgery. Such a book sets out the ideal. This book however has a different starting point: the clinical situation, with the ways things are; not how care *should be* given but how it *is* given. It is the authors' experience that there is often a major difference.

By looking at some aspects of the real world of clinical nursing and comparing common practice with research findings, we will show that vital areas of nursing are failing to reach the standards we expect for the latter years of the twentieth century. The result is that nursing care is failing the patient because it is institution- rather than patient-driven. The institutions examined in this book are the hospitals, the medical establishments and the traditions and history of nursing. Where these institutions dominate, the result is that nursing fails the patient and fails itself.

The cause of this failure, we suggest, is rooted in the traditional rituals and myths that still abound in the wards and departments of hospitals today. Chapman (1983) powerfully described ritualistic nursing practices relating to birth, death, status and power in her study of five large hospitals in south London. She discussed these actions not only in terms of defences against the stresses of the job (Menzies, 1970) but also as social acts which convey meaning to other nurses.

Ritual action implies carrying out a task without thinking it through in a problem-solving, logical way. The nurse does something because this is the way it has always been done. Perhaps actions have become enshrined in the holy tablets of stone known as the procedure book, or just: 'This is the way Sister likes it done'. Either way, the nurse does not have to think about the problem and work out an individual solution; the action is a ritual.

The mythology of nursing consists of all the stories that have little or any foundation in fact, yet such myths are a powerful force in everyday nursing. On the one hand there are myths about practical procedures such as dressings which lead to some exceedingly bizarre practices; on the other, there are myths about patients and people, which are stereotypes. It is a common feature of stereotypes that they bear little resemblance to the truth (Hildgard et al., 1987).

Thus, despite all the research that has shown that the best wound-healing environment is a moist one (Turner, 1985), why does a staff nurse spend 20 precious minutes twice a day hosing down and drying out a pressure sore with piped oxygen? Why do nurses base their assessment of the amount of pain a patient is suffering, and hence the analgesia they give, upon gender, nationality or type of operation rather than on what the patient reports (see Chapter 3)?

The staff nurse with the oxygen tubing in her hand has either not read any research on wound-healing or, having read it, chooses to disbelieve it in favour of the folk ritual or mythology of the ward. As we shall see, traditional nursing is based on many unsubstantiated beliefs, but not so many facts. Qualified staff who do not keep up to date with research findings have little other than intuition, outdated teaching, ritual and mythology to guide their practice. While there may be a place for intuition in the art of nursing, there is no place in the science of nursing for ritual and mythology!

An alternative perspective sees the nurse just carrying out orders from senior staff in the unquestioning tradition of obedience inherited as part of the Victorian legacy – with which nursing is still struggling today. This involves obedience to hierarchy and also to men, who, according to Victorian values, are seen as inherently superior to women. It is no accident that most nurses are women and most doctors are men. We shall return to this theme later.

In discussing nursing care and the application of theory and research, we can hear the reader asking: 'What about common sense?' The use of common sense involves working out a solution to a problem, not carrying out ritualistic actions, and to arrive at a correct solution the nurse must be working from facts not myths. Common sense is highly preferable to ritualistic action.

When considering factors such as pain we should look at patients as individuals not stereotypes. Statements such as: 'Men are big softies, they do carry on so' or 'After a small operation such as an appendicectomy the patient should only require one or two postop injections for pain' fail to recognize anything individual about the patient – they are stereotypes that have become part of the nursing mythology. In the following chapters we hope to explore the rituals of nursing that have become interwoven into a powerful belief system. We would like to set against those myths our view that nursing should be humane, therapeutic, democratic and adventurous. It should recognize the patient's basic human rights – freedom and choice – and we also strongly argue that such a choice can only be made rationally if the patient is in full possession of all the facts. The patient has the right to have knowledge and information, and the right to be fully involved in planning care, so that when consent is given, it really is informed consent.

We argue in favour of innovative nursing – nurses must recognize that they have a major role in the active rehabilitation of patients while still in hospital. This is reflected in the self-care philosophy of theorists such as Dorothea Orem; nursing must be prepared to let go of areas it has traditionally defended as its own territory in the interest of greater patient and family participation.

Our aim is to study a series of clinical settings and suggest how research evidence challenges practice. We will make suggestions for improving care in the light of research and in conclusion discuss why this state of affairs should have arisen. If the reader feels uncomfortable with some of the ideas expressed, we suggest you stop and ask yourself why. The basic question we ask is: 'Why should a profession behave so unprofessionally?'

It should be noted that, as the authors' experience is confined to general hospital situations, so is this book. However, areas such as mental illness and community nursing also have the same problems of unthinking ritualization and mythology.

REFERENCES

Association for Care of the Elderly. (1988). *Standard of Care Project*. RCN. Unpublished.
Chapman G. E. (1983). Ritual and rational action in hospitals. *Journal of Advanced Nursing*, **8**, 13–20.
Hildgard E., Atkinson, R., Atkinson, R. (1987). *An Introduction to Psychology*. New York: Harcourt Brace and Jovanovitch.
Menzies I. (1970). *The Functioning of Social Systems as a Defence against Anxiety*. London: Pamphlet no. 5. Tavistock.

Orem D. (1985). *Concepts of Practice.* New York: McGraw Hill.
Turner T. D. (1985). Which dressing and why? In *Wound Care* (Westaby S., ed.). Oxford: Heinemann.

PART ONE

The Rituals
of Clinical
Practice

1 Preparing the patient for surgery

Surgery is a medical intervention that can happen to a person anywhere between the first day of life and the last. After the skill of the surgeon and the theatre team, the next most important factors that will determine the outcome of surgery are the care given both pre- and postoperatively. Therefore we need to examine how much preoperative preparation is governed by research findings and care for the patient as an individual, and how much is ritual and mythology.

Preoperative preparation can be split into two broad areas — physiological (such as operation site, gastrointestinal tract) and psychosocial (such as giving information to the patient and family).

Physiological

'I know your operation isn't until tomorrow morning, but you cannot have anything to eat or drink tonight.'

Anaesthetists require patients to have an empty stomach in order to eliminate the risk of vomiting and inhalation during induction of anaesthesia and endotracheal intubation. From this essential requirement has grown the ritual of starving patients preoperatively for considerable lengths of time which bear little resemblance to the physiological requirements. This practice was researched and the problems it creates for patients were discussed as long ago as 1972 in an early Royal College of Nursing research study (Smith, 1972).

A typical morning list might have several patients and operating times spanning the period from 0830 to 1300 hours or later. All patients on that list will probably be starved from midnight. Thus the minimum period of starvation is $8\frac{1}{2}$ hours, while for others it may be over 13 hours. An afternoon list will probably require similar periods of starvation. If the operation of a patient towards the end of a list is postponed, he or she may then undergo a similar period of starvation the following day.

Alternatively in trauma surgery, where operating lists are less rigid than in a general theatre being shared by teams of surgeons, a patient such as an elderly lady with a fractured hip may find she is simply put on to the next list, extending her period of fasting to perhaps 20 hours. Given the unpredictable nature of trauma, such delays in operating times are inevitable.

This ritualistic starving of all patients for periods of between 8 and up to 20 hours poses certain questions:

1. How long is it actually necessary to starve a patient in order to empty the stomach?
2. Should all patients on the same list be starved from the same time, when this means that the last patient is starved up to 5 hours longer than the first?
3. Are there any damaging physiological effects from this lengthy period of starvation?
4. How does this affect the patient psychologically?
5. Are there more rational ways of ensuring that the anaesthetist's requirement of an empty stomach is met?

Let us start with the first question. Nimmo et al (1983) found that a light meal of tea and toast only 2–3 hours before surgery had no effect on the volume or pH of gastric contents. Work by Bateman and Whittingham (1982) demonstrated that 500 ml of fluid had a half-life of 22 ± 2.5 minutes and that a standard meal of 300 ml had a half-life of 64.7 minutes. (The term *half-life* means that half the volume of fluid would have left the stomach in 22 minutes, therefore only 250 ml would remain. After a further 22 minutes the volume remaining would be 125 ml. The same idea applied to the ingestion of a 300 ml meal reveals that after 65 minutes, only 150 ml remains in the stomach.) Finally we may note that Summerskill (1976) showed that peak gastric activity and acid output all occurred within the first hour of eating. Findings such as these about basic physiology seem to suggest that a 4 hour period of starvation is the maximum needed for any one patient.

The authors' experience suggests that 8 hours is the minimum starvation normally imposed and that much lengthier periods are common. Is there any quantitative research to back up our impressions? Reference has already been made to Smith (1972) who indeed confirmed such lengthy periods as the norm, but as her work was done before any of the research quoted above, have things changed for the better since the early 1970s? A replication of Smith's study by Thomas (1987) suggests that things are just the same.

In her study, Thomas found that patients on morning lists were fasted for a minimum of 10 hours with one patient being starved for 18.2 hours. Afternoon patients fared no better – the most unfortunate patient was starved for 22 hours! This is clearly a case of unthinking and ritualistic rather than rational action. It is made all the more interesting by the fact that the hospital in question had a 6 hour fasting rule – the first of many examples that we shall meet of a paper procedure that has little relevance to actual practice. The situation encountered here is that of a blanket rule applied to all patients on a list, regardless of where the patient is on that list and the likely time of surgery. Research shows that the time rule is probably 2 hours too long, but most worryingly when applied in practice, this blanket rule is leading to patients being starved for extremely lengthy periods.

While it may be argued that a day without food does the patient no harm – although psychologically it may be very unpleasant and a source of further preoperative stress and anxiety – a day without fluid intake most certainly is harmful, particularly to the elderly patient. It is possible that by the time patients reach theatre they are dehydrated.

Intravenous infusions (IVI) are traditionally started in the anaesthetic room, and may be run to cover the patient's metabolic requirements during surgery and in recovery. However the IVI regime probably does not take account of the dehydration that has occurred in the 24 hours before surgery, as the patient has had no fluid intake in a centrally heated ward; thus, fluid loss has been considerably increased by perspiration through the skin. The result is a patient returning from theatre in a dehydrated condition whose IVI regime does not recognize the preoperative dehydration that has occurred, no matter how carefully factors such as blood loss in surgery are taken into account. Could this help to account for the poor urine output, confusion and electrolyte imbalances seen particularly in the elderly after surgery?

Apart from causing avoidable physiological harm to patients, unnecessary fasting has been suggested as a contributory factor to preoperative stress. This is particularly so when nobody has bothered to explain to patients how long they must fast and why! The study of Thomas (1987) found that 76% of the patients were unaware why and 62% were unaware how long they were being fasted for. Instead they witnessed the removal of their water jug and glass, as if they were naughty children being punished because they could not be trusted to obey instructions. It is something of a mystery that having removed the jug and water, nurses always leave the patient's fruit or biscuits on the locker top. Perhaps the patient can be trusted not to eat, but not to abstain from drinking?

The work of many researchers such as Hayward (1975) has demonstrated that giving information to patients reduces stress and anxiety; in turn this has a beneficial effect on the amount of postoperative pain felt and recovery rates. It is highly likely that when we deprive a person of basic human activities such as being able to eat and drink, without a proper explanation why and how long this state of affairs will continue, we are denying the patient information, as defined by Hayward. This denial may hinder recovery just as much as the more obvious physiological dehydration inflicted on the patient.

One further aspect of this problem needs consideration. If patients are not told why and how long they are being fasted, the nurse is less likely to achieve compliance – the patient may eat or drink inside the forbidden 6 hours. If the nursing staff discover that the patient has broken the fasting rule the anaesthetist will order the cancellation or postponement of surgery as the induction of anaesthesia would be too dangerous. However, supposing nobody finds out and the patient goes into the anaesthetic room having just sneaked a glass of milk and a biscuit?

Fasting patients for longer than 6 hours has no basis in fact. The belief that such lengthy periods are needed is a myth. The blanket fasting of all patients, regardless of their position on the list, is a ritual which is detrimental to patient welfare. The anaesthetists interviewed in Thomas's (1987) study favoured working back from the patient's scheduled time on the operating list to calculate the time from when they were to be starved. Surely, as professionals with a creed of individualized, rational, problem-solving care, we should adopt this solution to the patient's problem?

We must also ensure that patients know why and for how long they are being fasted; if, for some reason, there is a delay which means that a patient will be fasted for a period of more than, say, 8 hours, then the medical staff should be requested to site an IVI immediately to ensure that the patient is kept well hydrated before surgery.

Recommendations for good practice

1. The starving period should be 4–6 hours.
2. This time should be calculated back from the scheduled operating time and individualized for each patient.
3. The patient should be told that he or she has been designated nil by mouth, why and for how long. This should be carefully explained

and then checked to see that the patient has understood. It is not what is taught that matters, but what is learnt.

4. Any patient nil by mouth for 8 hours should have an IVI.

5. A mouthwash to rinse out and freshen the mouth should be offered regularly during the fasting period.

'I've just come to shave you before your operation, Mr Brown.'

In order to minimize the risk of wound infection the operation site needs to be as free from microorganisms as possible. This basic surgical truth has led to much ritual in the preparation of the patient for theatre; one major example is the practice of shaving hair from a wide area of the body around the operation site.

This task is sometimes allocated to a theatre porter, often to a nurse. Much staff time is therefore spent in shaving patients, often in intimate areas, causing a great deal of embarrassment. The patient's skin may be cut accidentally, and he or she may suffer abrasions and soreness from the after-effects. A study by Winfield (1986) found that 22% of shaved patients had cuts or significant skin abrasions after preop shaving.

Various studies of the effect of shaving on the skin have been published. In the hours before theatre the abrasions and cuts sustained during shaving may rapidly become colonized by microorganisms, with the result that infection risks may have been increased, not decreased. Much work has confirmed these suspicions (Lancet editorial, 1983; Winfield, 1986) and the use of a depilatory cream to remove hair has been shown to be associated with a lower postoperative infection rate.

The American Operating Room Nursing Journal, in a draft updating of proposals for patient preparation (American Operating Room Nursing Journal, 1987) has stated that shaving is only acceptable when there is no time to carry out depilation by cream or if electric clippers are not available. If the patient has to be shaved, it must be a wet shave as this is much less traumatic to the skin than dry shaving.

In Winfield's (1986) study, those patients who used depilatory cream as opposed to shaving stated that they found it very satisfactory. Those who had previously experienced the traditional preop shave stated a strong preference for the cream. Winfield found that it often took several disposable razors to carry out a full shave at an average cost of 20–25 p per patient. The average cost of depilation was 50 p. When one considers the savings in staff time, however, coupled with the greater comfort and reduction in embarrassment for the patient, it makes more sense economically and otherwise to use a depilatory cream. Finally, if the use of cream prevented just one major postop wound infection in a year, its use would have been more than justified both economically and in terms of patient well-being.

In view of the overwhelming amount of evidence there is no place for the traditional skin shave as part of preop preparation. It is a ritual based on a myth.

We recognize that patient preparation is usually determined by the surgeon. In areas where such practices are continued, it is the duty of nurses, if they consider themselves truly professional, to assemble the evidence for change and approach the relevant hospital medical committee or, if it is more appropriate, to make an individual approach to the surgical consultant advocating change.

We have looked here in some depth at two major preop rituals. There are others however. Why do we remove all a patient's rings except the wedding ring? Are wedding rings in some way repellant to bacteria but other plain metal rings are not? Given that the ring may have remained on a person's finger for 50 years and never been taken off, why do we tape it on to go to theatre as if afraid it will jump off at the sight of a scalpel? If the purpose of the (non-sterile) tape is to prevent infection risks, then why not simply remove the ring along with the other jewellery?

The question of care-planning will be considered in detail in a later chapter (Chapter 15). However, in this section we must mention the paradoxical ritual of spending as much time completing a detailed nursing assessment form for a patient who is having an ingrowing toenail removed as for one who is having major bowel surgery for malignant disease. The completion of the assessment or admission sheet, as it is usually called, has often become a ritual devoid of meaning. How else can such a paradox be explained? A full discussion of this paradox – as much information is recorded about patients having minor as those having major surgery – will be given in Chapter 15.

Whether information recorded in this way influences the care given to the patient is another matter. How else can one explain nurses treating a patient for several days as a Hungarian who does not speak English, bombarding him with Hungarian/English cards and even a mystified Hungarian translator, when on his admission slip it stated under country of birth, Ukraine? Who had read the admission/assessment data before carrying out care?

Psychosocial
'But nobody told me about this before the operation!'
Reference has already been made to the importance of giving information

to patients (Hayward, 1975) admitted to hospital, whether for surgery or for any other reason. If nurses go about their work in a ritualistic fashion, it is doubtful that they will give patients the opportunity to ask questions. If questions are asked, it is likely that the nurse will avoid answering them, except in the most general terms or by reference to some other authority (such as: 'Ask the doctor').

There is much evidence to suggest that nurses are indeed prone to this sort of behaviour. A major study by Lisbeth Hockey evaluated how much information patients were given about mastectomy. In reporting this work, Anderson (1988) wrote of the greatly raised levels of anxiety amongst women in the time before going into hospital concerning their surgery and prognosis. Of the sample of 117 women in three hospitals, only 19% reported that they had been given information about the physical aspects of their operation. The same number felt they had been properly prepared to face the emotional reactions which accompany such major, mutilating surgery. The women in Hockey's study spoke most of the lack of information about how they would feel after surgery and what all the 'drips and drains' were for.

Only 11% of the women reported that they had had conversations with nursing staff centred on the mastectomy, as opposed to more social subjects and general chatter. Less than a third of the patients' relatives reported speaking to nursing staff at all; only six relatives of 117 patients actually discussed the patient's condition with nursing staff.

If we move from this study to more general areas of surgery we find the same pattern repeating itself. Summers (1984) studied a group of 40 general surgical patients and investigated their knowledge in the areas which had been identified by Hayward as contributing to a reduction in anxiety and postop pain (knowledge of the operation, probable time in hospital, preop preparations). Summers found that 80% of the patients scored 40% or less in a test of their knowledge. She points out that this implies that the patients had either forgotten or not been taught some three-fifths of what they needed to know. In carrying out interviews with the patients Summers felt that many of the areas where they were lacking knowledge could readily have been dealt with by nursing staff preoperatively.

Turning her attention to a sample of 40 nurses in the same unit, Summers found that only 27.5% were aware of the connection between information, anxiety reduction, pain and recovery rates while only 10% had actually read the work of Hayward. In this case, one is tempted to ask what 90% of nurses were basing their approach to preoperative care on. Could it be the myth that patients should not be told or that patients would rather not know the truth?

The myth that patients come into hospital not wanting to know what will happen is largely exploded by Hockey's work. In her study only a quarter of the large sample said that they did not want to know and that they would rather leave it to the professionals. The younger women in Hockey's study (aged under 50) were particularly keen to know.

The value of preoperative teaching and information-giving in patients who are to undergo stoma formation is underlined by Model (1987). She describes how nurses, faced with difficult situations and questions, get into a muddle because they want to say something to help the patient feel better. Laudable though this aim may be, it is often inappropriate as the patient must first be helped to work through his or her feelings and fears.

The almost kneejerk reaction of nurses when asked about distressed patients is to say: 'Reassure the patient'. This usually consists of bland words of comfort such as: 'It will be all right'. One could forgive patients for not being too impressed with such a banal answer when they are confronting cancer, knowing they are to have a section of their intestines removed and the remainder brought out through a hole in the skin to empty into a bag on the abdominal wall. Difficult situations are not a time for the nurse to hide behind ritualistic tasks, appearing very busy and thereby deterring the patients' unasked questions or giving the excuse: 'Sorry, I'm very busy now, I'll ask the doctor to see you later' when a question is asked. The 'busy-ness' of the nurses was commented on by many women in Hockey's study and seen as a reason for not being able to hold a conversation with them.

An important part of helping the patient to come to terms with illness is talking about it. The myth of changing the subject to distract the patient – 'Watch some TV, it will take your mind off things' – or the ritual of bland reassurance and question avoidance are sadly regularly still to be seen in wards.

The nurse will only help the patient by engaging in conversation in a meaningful way and giving honest answers. Survivors of disasters are best helped by being allowed to talk through their experiences (Haslum, 1989); in the same way, a patient facing mastectomy is facing her own one-person disaster. She must be allowed to express her feelings and come to terms with what will happen.

The ideas of Model (1987) concerning improving postoperative function by preoperative teaching are a logical follow-on from many studies which have investigated this area of care. Felton et al (1976)

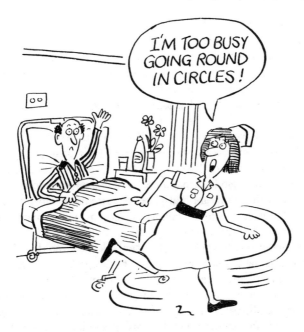

showed that in a study of 62 patients having major surgery for the first time, a structured preoperative teaching programme reduced anxiety and, measured on three different scales, produced a significantly higher level of psychological well-being.

Looking at the physical effects of preop teaching, we should consider a study by Fortin and Kirouac (1976); these authors took a sample of 29 matched pairs of patients undergoing elective surgery. Those patients who had undergone a preop teaching programme regained physical functional capacity much more rapidly than did the control group in ways which were not only statistically but also clinically significant. Like Hayward's patients, they also required a statistically significantly lower amount of postop analgesia and were discharged home on average 2 days earlier.

Johnson et al (1978), studying 81 patients undergoing cholecystectomy, again found that preoperative teaching reduced the length of stay in hospital and led to patients resuming normal activities more rapidly after discharge.

Studies such as these indicate that in our preoperative care we should not only be giving patients information in response to their questions, but also that we should have a carefully constructed preop teaching programme to facilitate postop recovery.

Such a programme is not as simple as it sounds, however; the findings of Nyamathi and Kashiwabara (1988) may tell us why, and also explain some of Summer's (1984) findings, discussed earlier. Nyamathi and Kashiwabara evaluated the effects of preop anxiety on the patient's ability to retain information and think constructively. Their study excluded cancer patients and those who had already been in hospital within the last 6 months; they only assessed those who were coming into hospital for day surgery. Despite these favourable factors, 25% had high anxiety scores on a questionnaire. When the patients were tested for critical thinking ability it was found that, as anxiety levels increased, so their ability to retain information and solve problems decreased. The implications of this work are that patients admitted to hospital tend to be very anxious and unless steps are taken to reduce anxiety levels, they will retain little information given by nurses.

We have seen that the belief that patients do not want to know what is happening to them is usually a myth, especially with younger patients under the age of 50. We have also seen that nurses tend to shy away from answering questions and becoming involved in difficult conversations with patients, hiding behind a smokescreen of ritualistic actions and bland reassurances. A mass of evidence shows that this behaviour is counterproductive to patient welfare; in contrast, spending time talking to patients, answering questions and working to an agreed preop teaching programme will help patient recovery. Nurses often say that they do not have time to talk to patients. We suggest that if talking improves recovery rates, it will tend to reduce workload and hence free the time needed! However we will discuss how nurses use their time later.

Recommendations for good practice

1. The ward should have a preop teaching package which is adaptable to the individual needs of specific patients and which should be implemented as an essential part of preoperative care.
2. Nurses should be encouraged to set time aside to talk to each individual under their care. Information-giving and anxiety reduction should be fundamental parts of nursing.
3. Nurses should be listeners as well as teachers. They should be encouraged to allow patients to talk through their problems and fears.
4. Have a periodic information audit on your ward to check how much information is being retained by patients postoperatively. In

this way ward-staff can evaluate the effectiveness of their preoperative teaching.

References

American Operating Room Nursing Journal (1987). Proposals for recommended practices preoperatively. *American Operating Room Nursing Journal*, Oct, 719–23.

Anderson J. (1988). Facing up to mastectomy. *Nursing Times*, **84**: 3, 36–9.

Bateman D. N., Whittingham, T. A. (1982). Measurement of gastric emptying by real time ultrasound. *Gut*, **23**, 524.

Felton G. et al (1976). Preoperative nursing intervention with the patient for surgery; outcomes of three alternative approaches. *International Journal of Nursing Studies*, **13**, 83–96.

Fortin F., Kirouac, S. (1976). A randomized controlled trial of preoperative patient education. *International Journal of Nursing Studies*, **13**, 11–24.

Haslum M. (1989). The psychology of disaster. In *Disaster: Current Planning and Recent Experience* (Walsh M., ed.). London: Edward Arnold.

Hayward J. (1975). *Information: A Prescription Against Pain*. London: RCN.

Hockey, L., Clark, M. O. (1984). Nursing research in Scotland. In *Annual Review of Nursing Research* Vol. 2. New York: Springer.

Johnson.

Lancet editorial (1983). *Lancet*, **8337**, 1311.

Model G. A. (1987). Preoperative and postoperative counselling. *Nursing*, **21**, 800–2.

Nimmo W. S. et al (1983). Gastric contents at induction of anaesthesia, is a 4 hour fast necessary? *British Journal of Anaesthesiology* **55**, 1185–7.

Nyamathi A., Kashiwabara, A. (1988). Pre-op anxiety. *American Operating Room Nursing Journal*, Jan, 164–9.

Smith S. H. (1972). Nil by mouth. London: Royal College of Nursing.

Summers R. (1984). Should patients be told more? *Nursing Mirror*, **159**: 7, 16–20.

Summerskill H. (1976). Measurements of gastric functions during digestion of ordinary solid meals in man. *Gastroenterology*, **70**, 203.

Thomas E. A. (1987). Pre-op fasting: a question of routine. *Nursing Times*, **83**: 49, 46–7.

Winfield U. (1986). Too close a shave. *Nursing Times*, **82**: 10, 64–8.

2 *The prevention of infection*

The battle against microorganisms has been a principle feature of nursing care since the days of Florence Nightingale and remains so to this day, particularly with the worrying development of resistant strains of bacteria and the arrival of the AIDS virus. In this chapter we shall examine three aspects of patient care to try and unravel the rituals and myths from everyday clinical practice and point the way to a more rational approach. The topics we will consider are dressing technique, catheter care and care of the patient with an IV line.

'Take Mrs Williams' dressing down just to see how it is getting along, Nurse.'

Patients who have returned from theatre with an occlusive dressing over their aseptically sutured wound are still subjected to the ritual of having their dressings taken down 'just to have a look'. Hopefully this practice is not as widespread as it used to be in the authors' training days (not that long ago!) but it still goes on.

There is no rational reason behind this act as it is possible to tell if there are signs of infection without removing the dressing, particularly if a transparent dressing is used. Pyrexia, redness around the wound, staining of the dressing, pain and tenderness at the wound site are all telltale signs of infection that can be elicited with the dressing in situ.

Thomlinson (1987) has pointed out that it takes 48 hours for a surgical wound to heal to such an extent that the skin has formed a protective barrier. Exposure of the wound within 48 hours of theatre therefore *increases* the risk of wound infection, and after the 48 hour period, as the wound is healing by primary intent, there is no point taking the dressing down because the wound is healing itself.

Wounds, in the absence of any signs of infection, should therefore be left alone to heal themselves. Taking the dressing down and swabbing with various antiseptic lotions before applying a new dressing is a ritualistic waste of time. Maybe this stems from nursing's obsession with tasks and the idea that being busy is the sign of a good nurse. If infection is present then we need to consider wound-dressing in a different light. Traditionally, a discharging wound is cleaned with antiseptic or normal saline and redressed at least once a day, sometimes more often. The techniques employed for wound-dressing vary enormously from hospital to hospital, yet each hospital teaches its procedure in a rigid, almost rote fashion, implying that this is the only way to carry out a dressing. The logical deduction from this is that everybody else is wrong and only we are right – clearly nonsense!

Aseptic technique needs to be taught in terms of principles. We are trying to prevent secondary infection of the wound during the dressing. This leads logically to the need to ensure that only sterile objects come into contact with the wound area during the procedure. As the nurse's hands are not sterile, this leads to a no-touch requirement, unless of course sterile gloves are worn.

The other two main principles are to prevent transfer of microorganisms from one patient to the other – cross-infection – and that staff must protect themselves from possible infection by the patient, especially with regard to blood-borne microorganisms.

A great deal of unnecessary ritual surrounds the way aseptic technique is taught. It is characteristic of nursing by numbers rather than of a professional, problem-solving approach based on logical principles. There is no need to waste time washing the trolley down before every dressing. If the sterile field of the dressing pack covers the trolley top and instruments are only in contact with this, what is the logic of even washing the top of the trolley, let alone the sides and bottom.

Nurses are required to wash their hands in various ways during a dressing; three hand-washes are not uncommon. Yet if the nurse's hands are not to come into contact with the wound, is all this hand-washing really necessary? If the aim was to make the nurses' hands free from microorganisms, then the full surgical scrub technique required of surgeons and scrub nurses in theatre would be required. If a lower level of disinfection is satisfactory, then the single use of an alcohol hand rub is sufficient, rather than multiple time-wasting hand-washing.

If we then consider the act of cleaning the wound with an antiseptic, there is immediately a problem in that the antiseptic will not be in contact with the microorganisms long enough to kill them. Thus the function of the solution is to wipe away the bacteria and other debris which may be a source of bacterial food; therefore an antiseptic is unnecessary.

The question of whether to use forceps or fingers to hold cotton wool balls when cleaning infected wounds was investigated by Thomlinson (1987) in a study of 74 discharging abdominal wounds. She compared the effectiveness of cleansing using forceps, a sterile gloved hand or an ungloved hand cleaned with Hibisol to hold the cotton wool balls. Results showed no difference in the effects of the different techniques, from which Thomlinson concludes that superficial discharging wounds may be safely cleaned by the nurse holding the cotton wool swabs with the fingertips of an ungloved hand, providing that a good hand-washing technique and Hibisol hand rub is used. Certainly, many nurses complain bitterly about the cumbersomeness of disposable plastic forceps, especially when in the interests of economy they are recycled. A cheaper, more convenient method is to use the nurse's hands. It must be emphasized that in deeper wounds or where there is a risk of blood-borne infection then the nurse must wear sterile gloves for protection.

The whole area of wound healing is a subject of much research and findings are systematically exposing much theory as myth and practice as ritual (see Chapter 3). Having already seen that antiseptics are unnecessary in conventional wound-dressing techniques, there is evidence from the work of Brennan et al (1984) that antiseptics such as chlorhexidine gluconate, povidone-iodine or desloughing agents such as hypochlorite solutions (e.g. eusol) adversely affect blood flow in the healing wound. The gains made in killing bacteria were more than counterbalanced by the losses in interfering with the wound healing process.

It is not easy to change from outdated dressing procedures based on myths and consisting of ritualistic behaviour which the nurse carries out without thinking about or without any insight into what she is doing. However, Ingleston (1986) has described one such transition which took 27 months to accomplish, using consultation and trials rather than an autocratic edict. In Ingleston's case, the wearing of face masks and cotton gowns, washing the trolley down before each dressing, the use of surgical spirit in wound cleansing and a triple handwash were all part of the ritual. Using a constructive, consultative approach, a more rational technique was eventually introduced, although it took over 2 years. However, it seems as if modern research is overtaking aspects of Ingleston's changes very soon after they have been implemented.

In discussing wound-dressing techniques there is one other myth that needs to be firmly quashed — the myth of the salt bath. Early work by Watson (1984) and Sherman (1979) had seriously questioned the use of

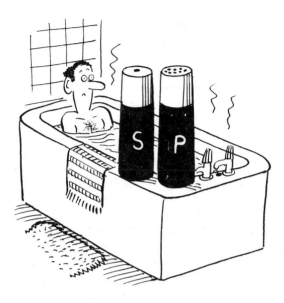

salt baths for healing or infected wounds. Both workers found large variations in both the amount and type of salt used, but could find no evidence to support the practice whatsoever.

Austin (1988) carried out a survey in a large general hospital. It revealed that 26 of 35 wards used salt baths to treat a range of conditions varying from infected or discharging wounds to incontinence rashes and pressure sores. The amount of salt used varied from half a cupful to three cups per bath. Given the differences in the amount of water that nurses might run into a bath, we can see immediately that there is no rational dose level or concentration being used.

Despite this nursing practice, salt is not an antiseptic. Aycliffe et al (1975) showed that adding 250 g of salt to bath water had no antibacterial effect and, in view of this, urged that the practice of salt bathing should be discontinued. Austin (1988) points out that in fact salt in solutions of up to 10% is used as a selective medium to grow *Staphylococcus aureus*, one of the commonest causes of wound infections! There also remains the possibility of cross-infection. Would you like to be the next in the bath after someone with a discharging rectal wound has been bathed?

Austin and others consider that salt baths have more to do with the psychological need of nurses to be seen doing something – anything –

even if it is of no therapeutic value. We support their view and urge nurses to think of their actions in a professional way. Confronted with much suffering it is not surprising that there is a strong urge for nurses to try something on the grounds that it might work. Nurses do not like to feel they are powerless to help patients. However we must balance these feelings against the evidence. Is there any research which supports the intervention that we have in mind? Could harmful side-effects outweigh any benefits? Only when nurses ask themselves questions such as these can they claim to be professional carers. Such an analysis must lead to the rejection of salt baths as another ritual founded on a myth.

Before leaving the subject of dressings, the impoverished state of the National Health Service forces us to look briefly at the practice of saving unused sterile dressings from CSSD packs. Roberts (1987) carried out a study of this practice on two surgical wards, with interesting results. On the wards studied, unused dressings from sterile packs were placed in boxes to be reused by staff as they deemed appropriate. Roberts took a total of 38 gauze swabs from the boxes at the end of 1 week. *Staphylococcus aureus* was isolated from 11 (29%) of the swabs; 2 of these swabs were resistant to penicillin and erythromycin, and the remaining 9 were resistant to penicillin only. Roberts points out that *Staph. aureus* is the causative organism in 18% of all hospital-acquired infections.

The worrying part of this study is that these unsterile saved swabs were normally used to cover and protect IVI sites and also to apply lotions and creams to skin. There is therefore a major risk of inappropriate use of these swabs leading to major cross-infection problems, particularly with penicillin-resistant *Staph. aureus*. The study concluded that while the two wards might save £60 per year between them in this way, the cost of treating likely ensuing cases of cross-infection far outweighed this minimal saving. The idea that saving unused gauze from CSSD packs might save money is therefore seen as a myth and a serious hazard to patient welfare.

Recommendations for good practice

1. Principles of asepsis rather than rigid, ritualized techniques should be taught. There should be a rationale for each action.
2. The practice of washing the entire trolley before each dressing is a waste of time, as is the use of masks and cotton gowns. A

plastic apron should be used to protect the uniform if an infected wound is to be dressed; it should be disposed of after use.

3. Wounds should be left covered and dressings should not be removed until the sutures are due to be removed, unless there are signs of infection.
4. The use of antiseptic solutions for cleaning infected wounds should cease; they should be replaced with sterile normal saline.
5. The use of forceps is not necessary to clean superficial wounds.
6. A dressing room should only be used to perform dressings if it is well ventilated and can guarantee eight complete air changes per hour. Otherwise, a build-up of organisms and cross-infection hazard will occur (O'Brien, 1986).
7. The practice of saving swabs from CSSD packs for re-use as non-sterile gauze should cease.

'Catheter care must be carried out according to the procedure manual.'

Many hospital patients have urinary catheters in situ for a variety of reasons. The management of incontinence by catheter however should only be seen as the last resort. Crow (1988) has carried out an extensive study of catheterization in hospitalized patients; her work shows that factors such as accurate fluid balance management in high-dependency patients and the facilitation of major surgery are two of the major reasons for catheterization.

The catheter offers ready access for organisms to invade the normally sterile bladder and set up a urinary tract infection which may ascend to involve the kidneys in advanced cases. Nursing care must then not only accurately monitor catheter drainage and ensure the patency of the catheter, but also as far as possible prevent urinary tract infection developing.

With this in mind health authorities have developed extensive and rigid procedures for their manuals concerning catheter care. Unfortunately, these procedures are rarely based on research but merely reflect the opinions of the author of the procedure – not a very sound base from which to conduct the battle against urinary tract infection. The picture is further clouded by the fact that staff usually ignore the procedure manual anyway! Crow's painstaking study of nursing care in several health authorities showed that nurses who followed the procedure manual were the exception rather than the rule.

Regular meatal toilet is a cornerstone of procedure manual catheter care. This action is carried out with a wide range of frequency, solutions and degree of asepsis. Unfortunately there is no evidence to support the value of any such intervention in reducing infections. Crow commented on this in her study.

Conti and Eutropius (1987) reviewed four major trials involving 2021 patients in the USA and concluded that none of the four care regimes reduced infection rates. In two of the studies, patients with meatal care had higher rates of infection than those who had no care at all, although fortunately this did not reach statistically significant levels.

These authors then reviewed the relative merits of latex and silicone catheters. Silicone is recommended for long-term use as body salts and other materials do not adhere to the walls of the catheter, so reducing the tendency to blockage. It was hoped that as a result there would also be less risk of infection developing, on the grounds that accumulations on the catheter walls readily harbour pathogens. However, a randomized trial found no statistically significant difference in infection rates. Silicone catheters are more expensive than latex but they do last considerably longer and are therefore the catheter of choice for long-term use. However their use on the grounds that they reduce infection risks has no basis in fact – it is a myth.

One practice which is gradually dying out is that of bladder irrigation to prevent infections. It has no beneficial effect and probably increases the risk of urinary tract infection as a result of the frequent disconnections of what should be a closed drainage system. Bladder irrigation may however be needed if the catheter has become blocked; a recent development aimed at avoiding the problem of contamination is the Uro-Tainer system. This consists of a prepacked sterile closed irrigation system which the manufacturers claim will significantly reduce the risk of introducing infection when a washout is performed to overcome catheter blockage. The manufacturers claim that the system may also be used to treat urinary tract infection. Independent research into the effectiveness of this innovation would be of great benefit to patients and staff in terms of quality of patient care and financial savings from a reduction in urinary tract infections.

The prevention of complications associated with catheters can be greatly aided if the catheter is correctly introduced in the first place. The appropriate size and length catheter should be introduced with a strict aseptic technique. The technique used by some members of the medical profession leaves a great deal to be desired. Nurses should always set the highest standard possible when catheterizing patients. Ritualistic measurement of urinary output which does not recognize the importance of fluid intake will be of little benefit to the patient. If the catheter is in situ, then the nurse must remember that output depends on input, and should therefore set a goal for fluid intake that will ensure good diuresis. A volume of 2–3 litres of urine per day may be expected to prevent urinary stasis in the bladder – a situation known to increase the risk of urinary tract infection.

Recommendations for good practice

1. The best way of preventing infection is by using a good aseptic technique when introducing the catheter.
2. Meatal cleaning has no demonstrated beneficial effect and is embarrassing to the patient. Continuation of this practice is therefore highly questionable.
3. Bladder irrigation with antiseptic solutions should not be carried out to reduce infection rates as it probably has the opposite effect. The cost-effectiveness of closed systems such as the Uro-Tainer should be evaluated in the treatment of blocked catheters.
4. Catheter bags should be emptied regularly and each patient should have his or her own jug to prevent the risk of cross-infection. This procedure is a potential source of infection to both nurse and patient and should be carried out with extreme care.
5. A good state of hydration ensuring a urine output of 2–3 litres per day will avoid urinary stasis and should minimize infection risks.
6. Silicone catheters should only be used for long periods. If a patient is to be catheterized for merely a few days, latex is just as good and much cheaper.

'Now hold on a minute, just a scratch in the back of the hand while I pop this needle in.'

Intravenous cannulation is a common practice in hospitals. Probably all patients have venous blood taken at some stage for analysis. A study by Krakowska (1986) recorded that 38% of patients in a typical week had either an IV infusion or a heparinized indwelling IV cannula. An IV cannula provides direct access to the patient's circulation, but it also offers a ready route of entry for microorganisms, the consequences of which may be infection on a systemic scale and the possible death of the patient.

A major European study (Nystrom, 1983) showed that 3.7 patients per 1000 acquired bacteraemia from peripheral vein cannulation while there was a 15.1% rate of thrombophlebitis. This study also found that 39.9% of surgical patients had IV cannulation − a similar number to Krakowska's study. Prevention of such infections is a major responsibility of both nurse and doctor.

Once again we find that health authority procedure manuals contain detailed step-by-step accounts of IV care and, as in the case of catheterization, one must ask what is the factual research base for such actions and, crucially, are they carried out in accordance with the manual?

Krakowska (1986) provides us with an illuminating insight into these areas in her study of a change in the IV cannulation procedure in one health authority. She found that 1 year after the introduction of a new procedure for the siting of IV cannulae, 40% of nurses admitted they had not read the procedure. Amongst a sample of 18 doctors up to registrar grade, none were aware of the existence of a hospital policy for IV cannulation. Observation of nursing staff and doctors during IV cannulation showed little adherence to the procedure; only 8% of doctors were observed to wash their hands unprompted before siting an IV cannula. This is borne out by the fact that in a questionnaire administered to the 18 doctors in this study, only 2 (11%) said that they always washed their hands before siting an IV cannula.

Such a state of affairs is probably not atypical. It calls into question the value of a procedure manual as a ritualistic, unthinking and unprofessional way of delivering care which meets with little compliance from staff. Only a third of the nurses interviewed in Krakowska's study felt that the new procedure was practical. We will return to the value of procedure manuals later.

The siting of an IV cannula is still largely a medical task in the UK, therefore detailed discussion of correct technique lies outside the scope of this book. Nurses are frequently asked to assist however, and it is important that the nurse should carry out her part of the procedure in accordance with the principles of asepsis (e.g. washing hands), not only for the sake of good nursing practice but also to set a good example to the junior medical staff who are frequently involved in IV cannulation. The nurse should also ensure that the equipment necessary for an aseptic technique is available. A well stocked IV trolley with a wide range of cannulae, blood sample bottles, and skin prep agents etc. should ensure that there is no excuse for the doctor to use an unsatisfactory technique.

Ward staff may consider monitoring the incidence of IV infections, thrombophlebitis and associated conditions, which would give valuable feedback to the medical staff concerning their competence. We cannot ignore the fact that Krakowska's observations led her to state: 'Doctors were assumed to be competent in the procedures required to put up intravenous infusions. As these results suggest, there is no reason to believe this is so'.

Once an IV cannula is in place, its care becomes the responsibility of the nurse, whether it is a peripheral or central line. Central lines have a greater potential for adverse patient effects, particularly if used for total parenteral nutrition, due to the ideal growth medium for bacteria. Nystrom's work, cited above, found that infection rates with centrally placed lines were 12 times higher than peripheral lines (44.8 per 1000 compared to 3.7 per 1000).

A study by Clayton et al (1985) found that *Staphylococcus epidermidis* was the infecting organism in 87.1% of infected internal jugular lines. The major cause of contamination was poor care of injection ports and three-way taps on IV lines. Speechley (1986) urges that stopcocks and three-way taps should be avoided in view of these infection risks and a major piece of work by Brosnan et al (1988) underlines the dangers of stopcock-introduced infections, quoting contamination rates of 46–58%.

With regard to the nursing care of IV lines, the need is for rational action based on research evidence. Actions should not be carried out because they always have been or because somebody thinks it's a good idea. Care should be based on preventing hazards that have been positively identified, as in the case of three-way taps and stopcocks, identified above. The patient's welfare demands that there should be no place for ritualistic action here, especially as many of these patients are very ill after surgery or on intensive care units.

Consider the length of time an IV cannula is left in place. Speechley (1986) points out that in view of research findings concerning the rate of colonization by bacteria and how the rate of bacteraemia rises with the length of time a cannula is in situ, an IV cannula should be changed every 48–72 hours. In Krakowska's (1986) study, the hospital policy was for resiting every 72 hours. However, as none of the medical staff were aware of the existence of any policy, it should not be surprising to learn that 61% of doctors stated they would leave an IV cannula in place until it fell out or until the clinical condition of the patient justified its total removal. Most of the rest of the doctors questioned thought that the IV cannula should be resited in under a week.

How active are nursing staff in documenting the length of time an IV cannula has been in situ and pointing out to medical staff that a change is now due? This would be a rational action in view of research findings, especially as, in fairness to medical staff, they cannot be expected to remember how long each of their patients has had an IV cannula.

In addition to the cannula, the giving set must also be considered as a possible source of infection. Most hospitals have policies about how frequently they should be changed, although there is no evidence to suggest that the recommended frequencies are adhered to, especially in general wards. This might make a fruitful area for investigation, as we suspect that many IV giving sets are never changed at all.

The Department of Health and Social Services (1973) recommended that all giving sets should be changed daily. Work by Band and Maki (1979) suggested that a 48 hour period is just as safe for peripheral lines; this recommendation has had effects on policy, particularly in view of the financial implications involved. The American Center for Disease Control recommended a 48 hour period for the USA in 1980. Recent reports indicate that a 72 hour change period may be equally as safe (*American Journal of Nursing News*, 1987). A study of 479 patients was reported to show no statistical difference in infection rates when peripheral IV giving sets were changed at 72 rather than 48 hours. The researchers urge more frequent changes however for blood products, total parenteral nutrition and arterial pressure monitoring, along with suspected cases of bacteraemia. They estimate that for their 450-bed hospital, this change will save $100 000 per year.

The financial implications of such savings should increase the pressure for change to less frequent intervals in the National Health Service. However, before such a change occurs, it is hoped that the research evidence will have been properly considered.

The dressings applied to IV sites vary from custom-made to home-made. A wide range of commercially made dressings are available, but many areas still rely on dry gauze and tape, with potentially disastrous results, as was noted earlier in this chapter. If the latter method is used, whatever comes in contact with the cannula insertion must be sterile. This is rational; rituals involving discarded dry gauze from other packs or pieces of sticky tape directly over the insertion site are detrimental to patient welfare. Independent research into the effectiveness of custom-made IV dressings compared with sterile gauze is needed: it does cost more to dress a site this way, but extra costs may be offset many times over if a reduction in infections can be expected.

Recommendations for good practice

1. IV cannulae should be changed every 48–72 hours.
2. IV giving sets should be changed every 48 hours. Research findings indicate that longer periods should be monitored.
3. IV insertion sites should have an occlusive sterile dressing.
4. Great care should be taken whenever a closed IV system is broken to prevent contamination.
5. Stopcocks and three-way taps should be avoided as far as possible.
6. Ordinary non-sterile tape should not be used to secure IV cannulae, but rather a custom-made sterile dressing.

References

American Journal of Nursing News (1987). News report. American Journal of Nursing 87, 1539.

Austin L. (1988). The salt bath myth. Nursing Times, 84: 9, 79–83.

Aycliffe G., Babb J. R., Collins B. J. (1975). Disinfection of baths and bathwater. Nursing Times, 71: 37, 22–3.

Band, Maki D. (1979). Safety of changing intravenous delivery systems at longer than 24 hr intervals. Ann. Internal Medicine, 91, 173–8.

Brennan S. S., Foster M. E., Leaper D. J. (1984). Adverse effects of antiseptics on the healing process. Journal of Hospital Infection, 5 (Suppl. A), 122.

Brosnan K., Parham A. M., Rutledge B., Baher D., Redding J. (1988). Stopcock contamination. American Journal of Nursing, 320–3.

Clayton D. G., Shanahan A. J., Simpson, J. C. (1985). Contamination of internal jugular cannulae. Anaesthesia, 40, 523–8.

Conti M. T., Eutropius L. (1987). Preventing urinary tract infections. What really works? American Journal of Nursing, 87, 307–9.

Crow R., Mulhall A., Chapman R. (1988). Indwelling catheterization and related nursing practice. Journal of Advanced Nursing, 13, 489–95.

Ingleston L. (1986). Make haste slowly. Nursing Times, 82: 37, 28–31.

Krakowska G. (1986). Practice versus procedure. Nursing Times, 82: 49, 64–6.

O'Brien D. (1986). Post operative wound infections. Nursing, 5, 178–82.

Roberts J. (1987). Penny wise pound foolish. Nursing Times, 83: 37, 68–70.

Sherman L. A. (1979). A pinch of salt. Nursing Times, 75: 45, 355–8.

Speechley V. (1986). Intravenous therapy, peripheral and central lines. *Nursing,* **3**, 95–100.

Thomlinson D. (1987). To clean or not to clean? *Nursing Times,* **83**: 37, 71–5.

Watson M. (1984). Salt in the bath. *Nursing Times,* **80**: 46, 57–9.

3 Lotions and dressings

In the previous chapter we discussed some of the mechanics of preventing infection. It now remains to look at some of the materials which may be used, whether on a pressure sore or a surgical wound. In the first section some of the agents used to clean wounds will be considered; then we will discuss the dressings.

'Pack Mr Johnson's pressure sore with Eusol and gauze, Nurse.'

In the previous chapter we considered closed surgical wounds which were either clean or infected and discharging pus. If a wound is open (such as a pressure sore) and containing black necrotic tissue, or deep (such as sinus wound) and discharging pus, different techniques are necessary. To promote effective wound healing necrotic tissue has to be removed and infection eliminated. One further requirement is that for complete healing the wound should close from the bottom upwards.

Over the years nurses have employed a large range of lotions and agents to remove necrotic tissue, combat infection and promote healing. Some of the remedies used verge on witchcraft and have as much to do with professional care in the 1990s as a cauldron full of newts' livers and bats' feet! This battery of remedies has its origins in the mythology of nursing. In the past a nurse would be told that an agent works and would, unquestioningly believe what she was told. That is how nurses were (are?) trained. The result is the propagation down the years to the present day of methods and lotions that are of no demonstrated value. Worse, some of these lotions have been shown to be positively harmful, yet they are still in use.

Nurse training has failed to produce practitioners with enquiring minds who ask: 'Why? How do I know that solution is of any value?' Sister says use Eusol so the nurse uses it and another unthinking ritual is propagated. Why does Sister say use Eusol? Because either she knows no better or because the medical staff have ordered its usage. Ritual and tradition are not the sole prerogative of nurses.

Eusol is a hypochlorite solution (others include Chloramine T, Chlorasol, Milton) used to remove dead tissue. There is a large body of evidence (Johnson, 1987; Ferguson, 1988) to show that its use should be banned for the following reasons:

1. Collagen synthesis is seriously affected because of the toxic effects on fibroblasts. Collagen synthesis is a key step in wound healing.
2. Serious damage is caused to the microcirculation; this will delay healing.
3. Endotoxins are released from the walls of coliform organisms when they are attacked by hypochlorites. These endotoxins damage the renal tubules and can lead to anything from mild uraemia to acute renal failure.
4. The effectiveness of these solutions as desloughing agents has been called into question.

If a new drug was brought on the market with these sorts of side-effects there would be an immediate outcry and it would be banned (Johnson, 1987). However because these solutions have been around for 20 years or more and given the ritualistic methods of nursing, they are still in use. The medical profession is equally guilty: how can hospital pharmacies continue to justify the practice of issuing these harmful and dangerous chemicals for use *against* patients?

The same arguments can be deployed against the practice of putting Mercurochrome on abrasions and minor wounds, yet the practice still goes on despite the fact that this agent was totally discredited many years ago. It delays wound healing by interfering with the normal physiology of healing and can lead to mercury poisoning if used over-enthusiastically (Goodman-Gilman 1980). Yet nurses in Accident & Emergency units still dab it on abrasions and hospital pharmacists still dispense it.

If we return to the question of removing slough and necrotic tissue from wounds, the answer is that any desloughing action that hypochlorites may have is more than outweighed by their many harmful side-effects. In the light of these known side-effects, a patient who suffered renal failure as a result of hypochlorite dressings may be entitled to sue the Sister responsible. There is little or no factual evidence to support the use of any other traditional desloughing agent, except perhaps the surgeon's scalpel. All that is left is anecdote and myth.

How then should wounds be desloughed? The evidence from carefully controlled trials points to the use of the modern substances which have come on to the market in the last 10 years.

The same answer applies to the question of ridding infected wounds of pathogens, a topic that needs consideration here. Once again the range of substances used varies from the bizarre (Marmite, honey, eggs etc.) to the predictable antiseptics. Putting aside agents that have no known antiseptic effect such as Marmite (however much the nurse may appreciate its flavour on toast) and concentrating on antiseptics we find problems. If they are used to swab superficial wounds, as we saw in the previous chapter, they will not be in contact with the pathogens long enough to kill them. If used to pack cavities, Johnson (1987) argues that they – particularly chlorhexidine and cetrimide – will be deactivated by pus and organic matter before they can kill many pathogens. There is always the risk of reactions and skin sensitivities (particularly with povidone-iodine), and antispetics may be toxic to the central nervous system if they come in contact with major nerves.

The use of topical antibiotic preparations such as Fucidin tulle is to be deprecated given the emergence of resistant strains of bacteria such as the much-feared MRSA (methicillin-resistant *Staphylococcus aureus*).

Whether we are dealing with a necrotic pressure sore or a deep, discharging sinus or wound, the implications are the same. Traditional methods fall far short of dealing with the problem effectively. Ritualistic dressing of the wound every day with agents when the only reason for their use is 'Sister says so' or 'We've always done it this way' is unacceptable nursing practice. Before looking at the available modern agents there remains one area to consider – the dressing itself.

'Just put a dry gauze dressing on that please, Nurse.'
Wounds need to be kept covered to prevent contamination and infection, hence the development of gauze dressings. However wounds need much more than simply covering, research has shown that the following factors are essential in the promotion of healing (Ferguson, 1988):

1. Excess exudate from the wound needs to be absorbed.
2. There should be a high level of humidity at the surface of the wound as epithelial cells require a moist environment to enable them to move across the wound surface.
3. There should be free gaseous exchange at the wound surface and the pH should be stable at around 6.1 for optimum healing.
4. No microorganisms should be able to gain access to the wound through the dressing.
5. The dressing should keep the wound temperature close to body temperature.
6. No foreign material from the dressing should be shed into the wound.

7. The dressing must be removable with the minimum of trauma so that newly formed tissue is not damaged.

It is worth considering some traditional dressings in the light of these findings, starting with the no-dressing dressing, in other words the practice of leaving wounds open. This practice clearly flies in the face of all logic and underlines the folly of nurses hosing down pressure sores with piped oxygen in the mythological belief they are hastening healing. They are in fact having the opposite effect by drying the wound out (Turner, 1970).

The traditional dry gauze dressing falls down on most of the points listed above. For example, gauze dressings are poor at preventing bacterial invasion, tend to shed fibres into the wound and can become firmly stuck to it, causing a great deal of trauma and pain on removal.

The use of non-adherent dressings (e.g. Melolin) is at least a step in the right direction, providing the non-adherent side is applied to the wound. Unfortunately the authors have seen wounds dressed with the non-adherent side facing away from the wound. This has led to companies introducing dressings with both sides made of non-adherent material. Such dressings are thin, and on their own insufficient to absorb any exudate. They therefore require backing with substantial amounts of gauze and the whole dressing must be changed as soon as exudate has soaked through, as bacterial invasion rapidly occurs through wet gauze. An alternative is to place extra gauze layers over the top of the dressing to prevent undue trauma to the tissue underneath, but there is a limit to the number of times this may be done.

Gauze dressings therefore are of limited value and in many situations are unsuitable. This leads us to consider the new alternative dressings that have become available in the last 10 years or so, and it is at this point that we may join together the threads of the discussion from the first part of this chapter with our current argument.

Firstly let us look at the infected wound or the wound with dead tissue surrounding it. A variety of agents have been developed that will deslough such wounds and also rapidly remove pathogenic organisms. They act rather like a vacuum cleaner, sucking out all the undesirable material from a wound; examples are Debrisan, Varidase and Iodosorb.

Johnson (1986) has described a typical successful trial with Debrisan, a substance consisting of beads between 0.1 and 0.3 mm diameter which is able to suck large amounts of fluid out of the wound, absorbing the exudate and swelling into a soft gel as it does so. Not only does

Debrisan absorb fluid, it also takes the pathogens with it, concentrating them away from the wound towards the surface, where they are observed to die quickly.

In this trial 60 g of Debrisan beads were mixed with 30 ml sterile Macrogel 400 to form a paste which had all the properties of Debrisan beads. This was used on a total of 18 patients with infected stasis ulcers of long standing. Within 5 days, 17 ulcers were free from any organisms; the 18th was still contaminated, but the organism responsible was also present in the patient's nose. This ulcer was seen to heal despite remaining contaminated with the patient's own flora.

The Debrisan treatment had eliminated the infecting organisms and left the wounds ready to heal. New products are expensive, and the cost may be raised as an objection. In this case it was estimated that a 5-day successful course of treatment cost £5.85, whereas conventional treatments would have cost £27.65, with no guarantee of success. Varidase may be used in the same way as Debrisan, is equally effective and may prove cheaper. It is also very versatile as it can be applied in several different ways.

Given that powerful new techniques are available to remove necrotic tissue and infecting pathogens from wounds and that these techniques are far more effective than traditional methods and, unlike some such methods, do the patient no harm, why are we not using them? Why do we remain in the land of lotions and potions, using solutions that are not solutions to problems? If clinical practice was rational this would not be the case, this suggests that we lack a rational base for nursing today.

It remains for us to look at the new dressings available. They have been designed to meet the criteria discussed above and come in different forms. One approach is to try and fill the wound cavity completely to promote healing from below; examples of this are foams (e.g. silastic foam), hydrogels (e.g. Gellperm) or fibrous products (e.g. Sorbsan). These should supersede the traditional wound-packing with ribbon gauze and eusol, povidone-iodine, Flamazine or Eusol and paraffin to name but a few examples encountered by the authors recently.

Another approach involves the use of hydrocolloids such as Granuflex and Comfeel Ulcus. These are totally occlusive dressings and again are very successful, particularly in dealing with difficult long-standing wounds such as pressure sores and leg ulcers. The ulcers referred to in Johnson's (1986) study were dressed largely with Granuflex after the initial 5-day desloughing and disinfecting period, and they healed rapidly.

Major trials have demonstrated the effectiveness of Granuflex (van Rijswijk et al, 1985; Cherry et al, 1984). As a small-scale example, Pottle (1987) has described the impact of Granuflex on a series of long-standing leg ulcer patients in the community who had had every conceivable traditional treatment tried upon their ulcers. One patient had been treated for a staggering 10 years at a calculated cost of £47,280 for a leg ulcer. Granuflex healed the ulcer in 6 months at a cost of £1282. Pottle found that Granuflex healed ulcers of many years' standing in a matter of months, or greatly reduced the ulcer size and, crucially, the pain and discomfort they were causing the patients. The initial phase of treatment was found to be associated with increased discharge and smell due to lysis of the necrotic tissue; patients needed extra support in this phase but once this was successfully negotiated healing continued at a rapid rate.

One final technique involves the use of films such as OpSite or Tegaderm which are highly suitable for treating superficial, extensive areas such as early pressure sores or burns. There is a problem in that these films cannot absorb exudate although this may be overcome by needle aspiration with an aseptic technique and covering the puncture area with a new patch of film.

An objection that has been raised to the use of such new dressings for the treatment of pressure sores is that they tend to slide off due to friction on the bedclothes, for example in the sacral area. As we shall see (Chapter 7), such friction is one of the major causes of pressure sores, therefore if the patient was being nursed correctly, shearing friction forces would not occur. The forces that tend to dislodge the dressing are the same ones that caused the pressure sore in the first place. The dressing will remain in place and the blood supply to granulation tissue at the base of the sore will be increased if shearing forces and pressure are kept off the patient's sacrum. The patient should therefore be nursed side to side, and even on his or her front if possible. There is nothing wrong with the dressing, only the nursing care.

The objection of cost has already been dealt with in the two trials discussed here (Johnson, 1986; Pottle, 1987). At first sight the new materials seem expensive compared with traditional gauze and solutions, but so did penicillin. It is false economy not to use the new methods. A rapid improvement in the patient's condition saves money and human suffering far more effectively than penny-pinching.

When new products are introduced nurses must use them in accordance with the manufacturers' instructions. They are meant to be used as directed because much time and money has gone into developing them to work that way. Nurses must beware the unsubstantiated myths that may lead to inappropriate use of products and even their rejection on unsubstantiated grounds that they do not work. To get the best from a product the makers' instructions should be followed rather than short-cuts and hunches. False economies should be avoided, such as trying to make one dressing do for two patients, since we saw in the previous chapter, that can lead to disastrous consequences.

Many nurses' practice of caring for wounds leaves much to be desired. It is outdated, ritualistic, and lacking foundation in fact or research. Such practice calls the credibility of nursing into question as a profession and is a rich vein of malpractice waiting for the legal profession to start mining on behalf of their clients. It would be sad if we have to wait until some health authorities or even individual nurses are sued before there is a major professional initiative to eradicate the scandalously low level of practice concerning wound care that exists in some areas today.

Recommendations for good practice

1. Hypochlorite solutions and Mercurochrome should be withdrawn from use immediately.
2. No agent should be used on a wound unless a well substantiated case can be made for its usage. Custom and practice or personal preference are not sufficient reasons.
3. Topical antibiotics should be withdrawn.
4. The use of gauze dressings is only appropriate in a limited number of situations. Health authorities should identify these cases and decide upon cost-effective modern alternatives for other wound types.
5. All nurses must recognize that they have a professional responsibility to update their knowledge on wound care in line with research findings and modern developments. Failure to do so should be considered a breach of the UKCC Code of Professional Conduct.
6. Nurses should follow the manufacturers' instructions when using dressings to ensure that the best results are obtained.
7. Quality control should include regular audits of the types and effectiveness of dressings used, and the techniques of the nursing staff applying those dressings.

References

Cherry G. W., Ryan T., McGibbon D. (1984). Trial of a new dressing in venous leg ulcers. *The Practitioner*, **288**, 1175–8.

Ferguson A. (1988). Best performer. *Nursing Times*, **84**: 14, 52–5.
Goodman-Gilman A., ed. (1980). *The Pharmacological Basis of Therapeutics*. New York: Macmillan Publishing Co.
Johnson A. (1986). Cleaning infected wounds. *Nursing Times*, **82**: 37, 30–4.
Johnson A. (1987). Wound care. *Nursing Times*, **83**: 36, 59–62.
Pottle, B. (1987). Trial of a dressing for non-healing ulcers. *Nursing Times*, **83**: 12, 54–8.
Turner T. D. (1970). In *Proceedings of Symposium on Wound Healing* (Sundell B. ed.) Espoo, Finland: Gothenberg Lindgren & Soner.
van Rijswijk L., Brown D. et al (1985). Multicenter clinical evaluation of a hydrocolloid dressing for leg ulcers. *Cutis*, **35**, 173–6.

4 Nurses, patients and pain

'The drug round is due in half an hour, just wait until then for something for your pain.'
Nursing care should be organized on an individualized basis, and many nurses claim that it is. However as we shall see (Chapter 8) many ward areas still use a classic piece of task allocation, the drug round, whereby at fixed times two nurses give out medication, including analgesia, to all patients on the ward.

How might this affect a patient who is in pain? Firstly it means that few patients will receive their medication from the nurse who has been caring for them that day and who hopefully has gained insight into their need for pain relief. Perhaps even more significant is the fact that to the patient it appears that pain relief is only available at fixed times of the day, rather than when the patient feels pain or even more crucially, *in advance* of when pain is felt. Pain is a continuing experience, it does not come and go with the times of the drug round.

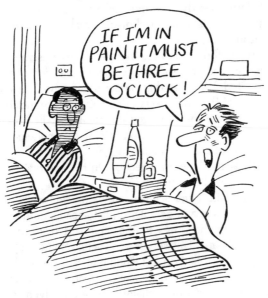

IF I'M IN PAIN IT MUST BE THREE O'CLOCK!

Sofaer (1984) has graphically described patients waiting for the drug round, lying in pain, yet afraid to ask for analgesia in advance. Patients may even be unaware that analgesia prescribed for them may be given at times other than the drug round. A nurse caring for a patient who has made his pain known to her, may on reporting this to the nurse in charge of the ward be told: 'I'll be round with the drug trolley soon'. Patients may feel inadequate if they ask for analgesia before the known drug round time and nurses by their attitudes have been shown to reinforce this feeling of inadequacy (Sofaer, 1984).

We can see therefore that a system usually involving one qualified nurse and an assistant giving out analgesia at fixed time intervals will not meet the patient's need for pain relief, neither is it conducive to the prevention of pain by giving medication before the patient's pain becomes a significant problem. In Chapter 8 we will argue that a primary nursing approach offers the best solution to the difficulties of the traditional drug round.

The statement that prevention is better than cure is a truism, but none the less correct. Consider the case of Mary Young, a 49-year-old lady who is recovering from a mastectomy. She asks the nurse for something to relieve her pain and the nurse, looking at her drug chart, notes that she may have 10–15 mg Omnopon 4–6-hourly. An intramuscular injection of 10 mg Omnopon is duly given. Half an hour later Mary is being violently sick and the physical effort of this adds greatly to her pain. Her psychological distress makes her wish out loud that she were dead.

At this stage the staff nurse notices that she is also prescribed 12.5 mg prochlorperazine i.m. and proceeds to give her an injection of antiemetic after she has vomited. Why has this happened? Because the staff nurse was either unaware of the side-effects of narcotics which include nausea and vomiting or because she or he did not think ahead to prevent the probable complications of the injection, giving the antiemetic at the same time as the narcotic. There again, maybe the staff nurse could not be bothered to draw up the extra injection. In the authors' experience, all three situations have been encountered.

The lessons are plain. Nurses must know the side-effects of drugs such as narcotic analgesics and be able to plan ahead. Another practical hint is to store antiemetic drugs in the cupboard next to the inner controlled drugs cupboard. This serves as a useful reminder to the nurse when drawing up a controlled drug. Planning ahead should also include consideration of factors such as when the patient is due to have physiotherapy or a major dressing change. Analgesia given correctly in advance may make these experiences pain-free and much more beneficial for the patient, as they can be carried out far more effectively.

Analgesia is usually prescribed in a flexible way, with a range of doses and frequencies of administration, e.g. 'pethidine 50–100 mg, 4–6-hourly i.m.'. This method of prescription acknowledges the variable and subjective nature of pain and there is overwhelming evidence from a variety of sources concerning the subjectivity of pain. It is a unique experience for each individual (Holzman and Turk, 1986), an experience that only the patient can feel. Given the uniqueness of the pain experience we can only agree with the views of McCaffery (1983) that pain is what the patient says it is and it exists when the patient says it exists. Given this latter point in particular, can we expect to deal with an individual's pain effectively with a rigid, routinized drug round? Such a philosophy contradicts the subjective nature of pain and the flexible approach to prescribing analgesia that is to be encouraged among the medical profession.

Let us look at some solutions, starting with a simple change to the drug round procedure. Being realistic about trained staff levels, it is probable that one qualified nurse will still have to do the whole ward round. However if the nurse responsible for each group of patients becomes the second nurse responsible for checking drugs with those patients, she should be able to advise the senior nurse about the analgesia requirements of her patients. In this way patients will receive medication based on the advice of the nurse who has been caring for them over the previous few hours rather than two nurses who may have had little contact with them at all.

An additional benefit of patient allocation is that the nurse is more likely to be able to identify patient anxiety and fear. There is a view that some patients complain of pain only to get attention. That begs the question of why patients feel they are not getting the attention they need. The fears and anxieties that lie behind patients' insecurity can be explored with a patient allocation system, leading to appropriate nursing interventions that might not be made if the patient was either labelled an 'attention seeker' or simply given an injection to 'shut him up'.

The nurse responsible for a group of patients should ensure that patients know how frequently they can have analgesia. Patients should feel able to ask freely for pain relief without being made to feel inadequate or a burden. They should not feel they are being judged in some way by the nurse as weak or a malingerer. They should not have to lie in bed watching the minute hand tick round agonizingly slowly to the time when they know the drug round is usually carried out. A patient has the right to pain relief when he or she feels the pain, not when the nursing staff decide to do the drug round!

If, due to the prescription times, it is not possible for the patient to be given analgesia for perhaps another half-hour, the nurse should think of other strategies to relieve pain, such as distraction or imagery (see p. 46), and be prepared to work with the patient to cope with that difficult period. It is clearly important in such a case that the medical staff should be made aware that the analgesic regime they have prescribed is inadequate.

Much work is now being carried out on patient-controlled analgesia which places the responsibility for pain control literally in the patient's own hands. Harmer et al (1985) describe the various options available, varying from the patient being able to self-administer a bolus dose on demand to patient-adjusted infusions – constant infusion plus bolus on demand or adjustable flow infusion plus bolus on demand. The technique involves the use of a computerized i.v. narcotic injection system which is under patient control but with built-in safety measures to prevent overdosage. While such a system is expensive it frees the patient from the wait for the next drug round.

Is the development of such systems an implied criticism of the quality of nursing care, indicating that nurses are unable to maintain their patients in a pain-free condition? An alternative explanation might be that such is the intensely personal nature of pain that it is impossible for another person to know an individual's pain experience, even an experienced qualified nurse. If the first explanation is correct it is a cause for concern, while if the latter case is true it is a cause for a little humility. We do not know as much as we think we know.

'After that operation you should only need one or two pain-killing injections.'

Hayward (1979) and Sofaer (1984) have both reported nurses associating certain types of surgery with preconceived ideas about how painful they should be and therefore how much analgesia they will allow the patient to have. Many researchers have found that patients suffer postoperative pain unnecessarily (Campbell 1977; Graffam, 1979; to name but two). There appears a clear link between these two findings if analgesia is being given according to the nurses' idea of how painful a certain operation or injury should be, rather than how painful it actually is to the patient.

The interplay of physical, psychological, personality, cultural and environmental factors which make up a patient's pain experience is so complex that no nurse can truly know what a patient is feeling. Giving analgesia according to the type of operation is the antithesis of the individualized care we claim to give and is potentially harmful to the patient as it may lead to unnecessary pain. Comments such as; 'Mrs Smith had the same operation as you 3 days ago and she is out of bed and not complaining of pain' are totally inappropriate, as Mrs Smith is Mrs Smith, not the patient in question. In addition they will only make the patient in question feel inadequate and possibly resentful of Mrs Smith. The pain experience is unique to the individual.

'If only the nurses had told me what to expect, but they always seemed too busy.'
A significant consequence of ritualistic practice, such as obsessional bed-making, is that patients never get the chance to talk to nurses; the nurses are always too busy. The result is that patients are unaware of what will happen to them after surgery. Hayward (1979) has clearly shown how information reduces anxiety levels and postoperative pain.

Many patients complain that they just did not know what to expect – how painful surgery could be and how difficult obtaining pain relief would be. These same patients often defend nurses by saying how busy they appeared to be, performing tasks such as making beds and cleaning cupboards. Nurses appear to withdraw from patients in pain, and focus their attention on ritualistic behaviour that has little to do with the patient. This may be seen as a stress reduction mechanism by nurses. Birch (1979) has reported on student nurses experiencing high levels of stress because they were unable, by virtue of their rank, to do anything to relieve their patients' pain. This sense of powerlessness was seen to cause the students to withdraw from their patients and avoid them.

Time spent on routinized, ritualistic tasks could be spent with patients teaching, informing and answering questions. This would help to reduce their anxiety and fear of the unknown, and consequently their pain levels. Building up patient relationships is a better use of time than cleaning cupboards. It is to be hoped that nursing reforms such as Project 2000 will produce nurse practitioners more skilled in the social sciences who will be able to recognize the importance of communication with patients and carry such ideals through into practice.

'You have to be careful giving analgesia in case the patient gets addicted.'
Nurses' fears of causing addiction have been frequently shown to be a reason for withholding narcotic analgesia (Graffam, 1979; Freidman,

1983; Saxey, 1986). In Saxey's study, 26% of nurses quoted addiction as one of the major side-effects of narcotic analgesia administration. Such fears are however unfounded in the case of postoperative hospitalized patients (Jaffe, 1975). The nurse may therefore give maximum analgesia as prescribed without fear of addicting the patient.

Addiction involves a complex interplay of social and psychological factors in addition to the pharmacology of the drug — factors which are absent from the hospital situation. Addiction as a result of a few days' administration of a narcotic analgesia to a postop patient is therefore extremely unlikely, but a great deal of pain may be caused if such drugs are withheld.

In dealing with long-term pain, two situations may be recognized. Firstly there is the pain of malignant disease which will become progressively more severe as the illness follows its course. Secondly there is the pain of non-malignant disease such as osteoarthritis. This latter type of illness is not life-threatening; the patient may have a life expectancy of many years and the pain is not increasing in the same remorseless way that is associated with cancer.

With non-malignant disease running a course of many years, repeated doses of narcotics may well lead to addiction and a case may be argued for avoiding narcotics in this situation. However for the patient with a terminal malignant illness, withholding adequate narcotic analgesia for fear of addiction is inhumane in the extreme.

A disturbing aspect of Saxey's research was the finding that almost 80% of the nurses interviewed did not know how narcotic analgesia worked. This finding is consistent with the work of Hosking (1985) who found that in a sample of 75 nurses, substantial numbers were unaware of the effects of narcotics. Is it surprising that many patients suffer pain when a large number of nurses seem ignorant of the pharmacology of powerful narcotic analgesics?

We may summarize the mode of action of narcotics as acting on the central nervous system to diminish the perception of pain and possibly also producing a feeling of well-being. Morphine given as an intramuscular injection of 10–20 mg has a duration of about 4 hours, varying with the individual. Diamorphine acts more quickly than morphine, but will wear off more quickly. Pethidine has an effective period of 2–3 hours before starting to lose its effect.

An understanding of narcotic pharmacology will greatly improve patient care. If a drug chart is written for the patient to receive drugs 4–6-hourly, then clearly the nurse must be monitoring the effectiveness of the drug well before the 6-hour period is up, given the short effective period of narcotics. Medical staff must be informed if the patient is experiencing pain before the prescribed time of the next injection. How else is the doctor, the only person who can change the prescription, to know what has been prescribed is inadequate? The nurse and doctor need to think whether the dose is too small, the timing not frequent enough or whether a different drug might be better.

'Pain is to be expected after an operation, so it will hurt for a few days.'

It has been demonstrated that many nurses believe complete pain relief after surgery is not possible and is therefore not part of their nursing aim (Saxey, 1986). Instead they think in terms of giving analgesia to reduce pain, not to prevent or banish it. Cohen (1980) has found that the amount of analgesia given to patients is much less than that prescribed by medical staff on an 'as required' basis (p.r.n.). Consideration of these two findings helps to explain why so many patients suffer pain which could have been avoided.

Medical staff correctly write prescriptions on a p.r.n. basis, leaving it to the nursing staff who are with the patients all day to administer analgesia as required. If nurses do not think it is possible to maintain the patient in a pain-free condition, or even see this as an aim for their nursing care, it is to be expected that many patients will suffer pain that could have been avoided. In Saxey's study, for example, monitoring vital signs and looking for haemorrhage were seen as higher priorities than pain relief.

It seems that many nurses will only give analgesia to a patient once he or she has developed pain rather than think of preventing the pain in advance by giving analgesia prophylactically. Are we guilty of thinking that the patient has to somehow 'earn' the injection by suffering pain for a period of time before we will give relief?

Nurses should use the freedom given to them by the doctor's prescription together with their knowledge of pharmacology and the individual patient they are caring for to make that person pain-free. Nothing less will do.

'I don't think Mrs Brown is in as much pain as she says; we'll leave it half an hour.'

Harriet Brown is a 65-year-old lady who has had rheumatoid arthritis for many years. She was admitted for an acute flare-up of her illness but now she is getting better and is sat out in the day room watching

TV with a magazine open on her lap. She has just told a student nurse that she is in pain. The student then received this rather dubious answer from the staff nurse. Why? On what basis has the staff nurse decided that .his patient, who has had many years to know how her illness affects her, is wrong?

When the staff nurse is questioned by the student as to how she knows the patient is not in so much pain, she points to the patient's observation chart. Pulse and blood pressure were normal when they were done half an hour ago. The staff nurse then goes on to point out that the patient's face does not show any expressions characteristic of pain, and anyway she is reading a magazine and watching the TV, so she cannot be in pain, can she?

In short, the staff nurse does not believe what the patient is saying in this instance. It does not occur to her that this patient has learnt to live with pain and adapt to it so that she does not display changes in vital signs or facial expression. Neither does it occur to her that Mrs Brown believes that you should not make a fuss when you are in pain. The staff nurse has not considered that Mrs Brown has learnt that watching TV or reading distracts her attention from the pain, making it more tolerable.

It seems trained nurses often fall into this trap and as a result set the wrong example to students as regards pain assessment. This highlights the importance of assessment in nursing care, for if nurses fail to recognize the patient's pain, they will be unable to intervene to relieve that pain. Jacox (1979) found that nurses pay little attention to verbal reports of pain from patients, rating them fifth out of a series of seven measures they would use to assess pain. Saxey also found that despite the statement 'pain is what the patient says it is', nurses in her study paid little attention to verbal reports of pain from patients.

The nurses in these two studies preferred to rely on physiological measures such as raised blood pressure or the appearance of the patient; facial expression or posture were favoured signs. However, the absence of a pained expression or posture does not mean the patient is free of pain; he or she may simply be using coping mechanisms to conceal the pain. Reliance on physiological measurement is also unreliable as vital signs may vary due to a whole host of reasons other than pain, such as anxiety or cardiovascular pathology.

Support for this view comes from the work of Camp and O'Sullivan (1987) who studied the pain experiences of 84 patients and how nursing staff documented their pain. The researchers found that less than 50% of the patients' reported pain had been documented, concluding that either nurses had failed to correctly assess the patients' pain and/or had failed to record it correctly. It is pointed out by Camp and O'Sullivan that law suits have been found in the patient's favour in US courts due to lack of correct, pain-related, nursing documentation.

A crucial element of assessment is recording the information for the benefit of future staff in such a way that it can be used to plan care rationally. Verbal reports of pain can easily be translated into an objective measure by asking the patient to rate the pain. Examples include the use of a numerical scale from 1 to 10 or giving a choice of five phrases to describe the pain in increasing severity from 'no pain' to 'most severe imaginable'. Repeated assessments of pain using such a technique allows nursing staff to see how effective their care is in relieving pain. When other information is recorded about, for example, the location and type of pain, this should assist in planning future pain-relieving care.

Factors such as culture and gender will also influence how pain is expressed just as much as the pain itself. The traditional British 'stiff upper lip' is a good example, contrasting sharply with other cultures where a freer expression of feelings is permitted.

Not only will these cultural factors affect how pain is expressed, but within the nurse they will also affect how patient pain is perceived. Davitz and Davitz (1985) found evidence of wide variations in pain ratings between nurses of different cultures. In their study British nurses assessed the amount of pain suffered lower than did nurses of any other nationality. The authors supplied anecdotal evidence to suggest that in American hospitals, British nurses were always thought of as very efficient but lacking in sensitivity to the individual needs of patients compared with nurses from other countries.

A similar study carried out by Taylor et al (1983) on hypothetical patients found that nurses attributed less pain to patients who had no obvious signs of pathology or who were suffering from long-term pain. Once again we see nurses deciding how much pain a patient has, based on measures other than what the patient actually says. The implication for good nursing practice is that when patients say they have pain, nurses should believe them!

A word of caution should be inserted here however. Some patients will try and disguise their pain in response to questioning, no matter how sympathetically it is carried out. Pain that may have been present for a long time may be coped with to such an extent that the patient will not admit that it is present. Jacox (1979) showed in her work that many patients did not like to talk about their pain; some two-thirds stated that they coped with their pain by silence. The nurse must therefore actively seek verbal information from patients about their pain, rather than waiting for the patient to initiate an exchange of information. The work of Jacox suggests that the majority of patients will not ask for analgesia of their own accord. The commonest reason amongst long-term patients was the fear of being stigmatized by nursing staff.

'You've only had a small operation so it shouldn't be that painful.'
Statements like this reflect the myth that pain is in some way linked to the volume of tissue involved. In fact the amount of pain is often unrelated to the size of wound or the extent of injury.

A classic study by Beecher (1956) of combat casualties from World War II showed that wounded soldiers consistently reported less pain than civilian patients. The former group viewed hospital with relief. They were just glad to be alive, while civilians had negative feelings about illness and hospital. There are many anecdotal stories of wounded servicemen performing heroic actions, seemingly without concern for the horrific injuries they had sustained. Nurses in the field of Accident & Emergency must have seen patients with severe injuries and yet little apparent pain, and inevitably compared such patients to others with minor abrasions or sprains who complained far more forcibly about pain.

Having emphasized the importance of assessing the degree of pain that a patient is experiencing, we must also try and find out what sort of pain is being felt. Consider the patient known to one of the authors who walked into Accident & Emergency complaining of bad toothache. When carefully questioned by the author at the reception desk he admitted that the pain was not localized to one tooth but affected the whole side of his face, the left side. Come to think of it, he had not been feeling well all evening and he had some funny tingling sensations in his left arm and a further question revealed his chest felt a bit tight as well. Five minutes later an electrocardiogram had revealed a myocardial infarction and within 25 minutes of going to Accident & Emergency complaining of toothache the patient was on the coronary care unit!

The lesson for all of us is that we must believe the patient who says he or she has pain, but we must also probe further and find out where the pain is, its duration and nature (tight, gripping, colicky, a dull ache etc.) and how the patient feels in general. If we had taken the approach that toothache only produces a certain amount of pain which could be controlled with over-the-counter analgesics such as paracetamol, the patient quoted above suffering an acute myocardial infarction might have been given low priority for treatment.

The nurse must understand the different types of pain experienced by patients and their possible clinical significance. Assessment must include more than just the degree of pain.

'She is not in much pain so I don't think she is suffering that much.'

The assumption in this statement is that suffering is in some way closely linked to pain. This is challenged by Kahn and Steeves (1986) who consider suffering to be different from pain. They consider it is an individual's experience of threat to self and the meaning the individual gives to events such as pain or loss. Suffering then is only partially dependent upon pain.

Thus a pain that might be otherwise easily endured will cause suffering if the patient imagines it will continue for a long time or get worse, or that it is a symptom of cancer. Conversely, the pain of childbirth may not be construed as suffering by many women because of the meaning attached to it and the knowledge that it is finite – there is an ending to the pain.

The ideas of Kahn and Steeves – that suffering is an experiential meaning given by patients to events such as pain – have a major implication for nurses trying to assess a patient's suffering. This presents the nurse with the problem of trying to interpret and understand the meaning of another person's experience. The nurse needs time, communication and empathy to achieve this, rather than ritualistic practice. A medical diagnosis and the nurse's view of how much it ought to hurt are no guide to patient suffering.

'I cannot give you anything for pain as your next injection is not due for another half-hour.'

So far we have concentrated on analgesia as a means of relieving pain. In her study, Saxey (1986) found that only a small number of nurses thought there was anything else they could do to relieve pain other than give drugs. The authors have also had this experience in working with students!

The interplay between anxiety and pain has been highlighted by many of the researchers referred to in this chapter, with the clear message to nurses that if you reduce anxiety, you reduce pain. Simply talking to the patients, allowing them the room and time to express their feelings and ask the questions they have been mulling over in their minds will make a major contribution to anxiety reduction.

Fear of the unknown is a major source of anxiety. What is familiar to the nurse working every day in hospital may be totally alien to the patient, and we should never lose sight of this fact. Consider how much patients understand of what they are told by doctors and nurses. A vague statement about a patch of inflammation in the bowel from a doctor may convince a patient that he has cancer. Such are the fears and anxieties which often make up a patient's day. Nurses must learn to communicate with their patients and to see teaching and listening as integral parts of nursing care, rather than as vague concepts they have to remember to write about to keep the examiners happy when they are students.

There are many nursing interventions which do not require a medical prescription, but which reduce pain significantly. We have already seen how information-giving reduces both pain and anxiety, yet Fagerhaugh and Strauss (1977) found that medical and procedural tasks were given a higher priority by nurses than the psychosocial needs of patients. If the quality of care is to be improved, much greater emphasis must be paid by nurses to the less task-oriented aspects of care, for although it is over a decade since Fagerhaugh and Strauss's work, there is still much validity in their findings. Qualified nurses can help redress this balance by the example they set students as they go about their care.

Nurses should consider how they can work with patients who have evolved their own coping mechanisms to distract their attention from chronic pain. In addition to distraction, the technique of imagery may be taught to patients. This involves imagining specific pleasurable experiences, such as the view from the summit of Great Gable, and describing what can be seen, smelt or heard. An alternative approach involves using images of pain seen flowing away from the body. The aim is to make the patient less aware of the pain.

Relaxation techniques also have a valuable role to play in relieving patient pain. Wallace (1987) has described the use of such alternatives to analgesia in a group of 32 women with lower pelvic pain. Each woman had been investigated by a gynaecologist and no significant pathology had been found. A control group from within the sample of 32 received no further active intervention but the other women were treated by relaxation therapy, behavioural counselling and psychotherapy. Over a 1-year follow-up period Wallace found that all the women who had been given therapy reported more pain-free days than the control group, and that relaxation techniques produced the best results of all.

Relaxation does not require a medical prescription but it does involve a large amount of patient involvement. This is beneficial as it helps the patient to feel that he or she is exercising control over both body and illness, and thus helps improve morale and self-concept.

There are of course many other ways of relieving pain such as massage, the use of heat or cold, alterations in position and splintage and elevation for injured limbs. Not all methods will work for all patients due to the subjective nature of pain. The nurse must be prepared to experiment with the patient to find the methods that work best for each individual. This is what is meant by individualized patient care.

In this chapter we have looked at conscious adult patients. The nurse should consider at least two other types of patient — young children and patients on intensive care. A young child has not developed the cognitive processes to handle such concepts as pain and therefore cannot respond meaningfully to questions about how much pain he or she may have (Beales, 1986). Different approaches have to be used which the child can understand (Burr, 1987), such as shading in drawings of the body with different coloured pencils. The more painful an area is, the more red the child is encouraged to use; less pain is shown by orange or yellow.

The patient who is being ventilated on intensive care cannot speak, so if, as we have been repeating, pain is what the patient says it is, that clearly poses a major problem to the intensive care nurse. Developments in ventilation techniques such as intermittent mechanical ventilation mean that heavy sedation and muscle relaxants are no longer needed for efficient ventilation in many cases. Many patients are therefore much more aware of their surroundings and able to communicate with nursing staff by means such as pointing. The use of a pain-measuring scale is therefore quite feasible with many intensive care patients.

Because a person is unresponsive does not necessarily mean that he or she is unaware of stimuli such as pain. This leaves the nurse in a very difficult situation when caring for patients who have, for example, suffered brain injury. However unresponsive patients may appear, there is always uncertainty about how much they may be aware of, and consequently, how much pain they may be feeling. Consider the work of Bergbom-Engberg et al (1988) who showed that, of a sample of 304 patients who were ventilated on the intensive treatment unit, 52% were able to recall the various treatments involved with their respiratory management — most in great detail.

Recommendations for good practice

1. Only the patient knows what his or her pain is like. Therefore the most important aspect of pain assessment is to ask the patient.

2. The use of pain charts will allow accurate documentation of pain which should facilitate effective nursing intervention.
3. Nursing staff should aim for a pain-free patient at all times, using pain prevention wherever possible.
4. Wards should carry out analgesia audits. Periodically, there should be a review of the proportion of p.r.n. analgesia which is actually being given to patients. If only a small proportion of the analgesia available is being given, are doctors overprescribing or are nurses underadministering?
5. Attention should be paid to the psychological dimension of pain. Relief of anxiety should lead to a reduction in pain.
6. Alternative therapies such as relaxation should be encouraged.
7. The nurse assigned to a patient for a shift should be involved in drug administration to that patient.

References

Beales J. G. (1986). Cognitive development and the experience of pain. *Nursing*, 3, 408–10.
Beecher H. K. (1956). Relationship of significance of wound to pain experienced. *Journal of the American Medical Association*, 161, 1609–13.
Bergbom-Engberg I., Hallenberg B., Wickstrom I. (1988). A retrospective study of patients' recall of respiratory treatment. *Intensive Care Nursing*, 4, 56–61.
Birch J. (1979). The anxious learners. *Nursing Mirror*, 149: 5, 17–22.
Burr S. (1987). Pain in childhood. *Nursing*, 3, 890–5.
Camp L. D., O'Sullivan P. S. (1987). Comparison of medical, surgical and oncology patients' description of pain and nurses' documentation of pain assessments. *Journal of Advanced Nursing*, 5, 593–8.
Campbell D. (1977). The management of postoperative pain. In *Pain, New Perspectives in Measurement and Management* (Harcus A. W., Smith R., Whittle B. eds.). Edinburgh: Churchill Livingstone.
Cohen F. L. (1980). Post surgical pain relief: patient status and nurse medication. *Pain*, 9, 265–74.
Davitz L., Davitz J. (1985). Culture and nurses' inferences on suffering. In *Perspectives on Pain* Copp L. A., (ed.) Edinburgh: Churchill Livingstone.
Fagerhaugh S. Y., Strauss A. (1977). *Politics of Pain Management: Staff–Patient Interaction*. California: Addison-Wesley.
Freidman F. (1983) PRN analgesics: controlling the pain or controlling the patient. RN, 46, 67.
Graffam S. (1979). Nurse response to patients in pain. *Nursing Leadership*, 2, 23–5.
Harmer M., Rosen M., Vickers M. D. (1985). Patient controlled analgesia. Oxford: Blackwell Scientific Publications.

Hayward J. (1979). Information: a prescription against pain. London: Royal College of Nursing.

Holzman A. D. (ed.) (1986). *Pain Management*. Oxford: Pergamon Press.

Hosking J. (1985). Pain relief: knowledge and practice. *Nursing Mirror*, **160**: 5 (suppl), ii–vi.

Jacox A. K. (1979). Assessing pain. *American Journal of Nursing*, **79**, 895–900.

Jaffe J. H. (1975). Drug addiction and drug abuse. In *Pharmacological Basis of Therapeutics* (Goodman L. S., Gilman A.) New York: Macmillan.

Kahn D., Steeves R. (1986). The experience of suffering: conceptual clarification and theoretical definition. *Journal of Advanced Nursing*, **11**, 623–31.

McCaffery M. (1983). Nursing the patient in pain. London: Harper & Row.

Saxey S. (1986). Nurses' response to post-op pain. *Nursing*, **3**, 377–81.

Sofaer B. (1984). Pain: a handbook for nurses. London: Harper & Row.

Taylor A. G., Skelton J., Butcher J. (1983). Duration of pain condition and physical pathology: determinants of nurses' assessments of patients in pain. *Nursing Research*, **33**, 4–8.

Wallace L. (1987). Chronic pelvic pain. *Nursing Times*, **83**: 50, 45–7.

5 Making observations

'Doing the obs' is one of the great time-consuming tasks of the nursing day. Consequently, nurses need to ask themselves just how frequently and reliably observations are carried out. Further, should they be observing more than just vital signs and if so, what else might come under the umbrella of nursing observations? In view of the great deal of time consumed by observations, their value and reliability are rightly the target of careful scrutiny. In addition, observation is synonymous with assessment, which is essential to nursing, for without assessment there can be no rational, individualized nursing care. We therefore need to investigate what element of ritual practice there is in 'doing the obs'.

'But that's the fourth time today you've taken my temperature and I feel quite OK.'

An elevation in temperature is part of the normal inflammatory response and consequently is associated with an infective process. Patient temperature is therefore one general indication of the presence of an infection, although there are many other symptoms or signs – some general, some localized.

If we first of all consider how frequently temperatures are taken, we find many patients on either twice-daily or 4-hourly recordings who have normal temperatures. Whilst frequent monitoring in cases of pyrexia or hypothermia is essential, the practice of taking the temperature more than once a day in apyrexial patients is a waste of nursing time, unless other observations make the nurse suspect that an infection or hypothermia may be present.

Samples et al (1985) examined this question from the point of view of the circadian rhythm that is present in body temperature. Its effect is to produce a maximum body temperature between 1700 and 1900 hours, making this the most sensitive time to detect any pyrexia. Much work cited by the authors in America has led to temperature recordings which are screening for pyrexia to be made daily, at this time only.

The researchers studied a sample of 107 patients, monitoring their temperatures over a 24-hour period. They confirmed the finding that body temperature is at a natural circadian peak around 1800 hours. They concluded that daily observations carried out at this time were sufficient to screen for developing pyrexia, unless the nurse observed signs or symptoms at other times which were suggestive of infection. Why then are apyrexial patients having temperature observations carried out between two and six times per day? Ritualistic practice appears to have taken over from thinking rational care. It is usually junior students who take the patient's temperatures and it is tempting to wonder how much their training has already conditioned them into unthinking obedience to orders. If the observation chart says '4-hourly obs' do students carry out these observations without thinking whether they are really necessary? If this is so, then clinical nurses and educationalists must shoulder the blame for not encouraging students to think and question.

A primary nursing system used by nurses who have been taught to take a questioning approach might prevent these situations, as the nurse allocated to the patient would constantly be updating the care plan. However, that nurse must realize the significance of the findings discussed above before common sense can prevail and temperature observations can be carried out at a more appropriate frequency. Similar comments apply to the frequency with which blood pressure, pulse and respiratory rate are recorded.

Having established the optimal frequency and timing of temperature observation, it now remains to consider how long the thermometer should be in place. Usual practice indicates that there is no fixed time; nurses leave thermometers in situ for as long as they feel like. This is a very unscientific way of measuring a vital sign such as temperature.

A study by Wintle (1988) found that the average time students left thermometers in a patient's mouth was 1.5 minutes, but there was a great deal of variation between first- and third-year students, with the more senior students taking shorter periods of time than first-years. In her observations, Wintle noted that students actually put the thermometer in the patient's mouth, recorded blood pressure and pulse, then took the thermometer out again to note temperature. As senior students were more experienced in blood pressure recordings they tended to be quicker, hence the shorter times for temperature readings. In practice students tend to leave the thermometer in place for however long it takes to record blood pressure and pulse − a practice which experience suggests they carry into their careers as qualified nurses. In view of Wintle's observations, it is tempting to ask if many thermometers are left in situ for more than 1.5 minutes if a qualified member of staff takes the temperature; if a student is involved, 2 minutes seems the likely time.

Can research give nursing any answers to the question of how long it takes to record a temperature orally? It is easy to determine how long it takes for a glass-in-mercury thermometer to reach a final reading, but a more practical question is, how long does it take to reach a clinically significant reading? For example, leaving the thermometer in the mouth for an extra 5 minutes might raise the recorded temperature 0.1°C, but is this significant in terms of diagnosing pyrexia? The patient's temperature might be recorded as 37.8°C, not 37.7°C, but is there any significance in that 0.1°C difference?

Closs (1987) examined the recommendations in 27 nursing textbooks and found times ranging from 1 to 10 minutes suggested by the various authors, only one of whom based the time on research. This subjective approach to measurement of such a vital sign is a very depressing symptom of much of nursing's mythology. When standard textbooks perpetrate myths, it is difficult to be too critical of staff whose care incorporates myths.

The response time of a thermometer in an experimental warm-water bath is 0.5 min, i.e. it will reach a temperature of 37°C in that time. In the patient's mouth, however, due to a variety of factors it takes considerably longer. A series of studies cited by Closs (1987) showed that a mean time of 12 minutes was needed to record maximum temperature. In an attempt to be more practical, the concept of optimum temperature was introduced. This is defined as the temperature reached by 90% of the subjects in these trials which was 0.1°C below their maximum. This was attained in 8 minutes by men and 9 minutes by women.

Other factors can of course affect the recorded temperature; the degree of error may be greater than the error due to the thermometer not being left in the mouth long enough. In her survey of 27 textbooks, Closs (1987) found only 2 that clearly stated that the sublingual pockets must be used to record temperature, as these place the thermometer in closest contact with arterial blood, and it is the temperature of arterial blood which we desire to measure. Failure to locate the thermometer in either pocket can lead to errors of up to −1.7°C in recorded temperature. Hot and cold drinks have also been shown to affect temperatures over a range from 1°C above to 3°C below actual temperature (Forster et al, 1970; Lee and Atkins, 1972).

Respiratory rate will affect temperature, even if the patient endeavours to keep the mouth closed. An interesting study by Durham et al (1986) suggested that patients with a respiratory rate above 20 breaths/min will have a temperature on average 0.3–0.4°C below those with a more normal respiratory rate of under 20 breaths/min.

The practice of recording rectal temperature in babies was examined by Kunnel et al (1988) in a study of 99 1–4-day-old normal neonates. Comparing rectal, axillary, femoral and skin–mattress sites, they found there was no difference in the final recorded optimal temperatures. However the rectal site took 5 minutes, axillary and femoral sites 11 minutes and the skin–mattress site 13 minutes to reach optimal levels. These differences were statistically significant and point out the wide variations in recorded temperature that can occur in infants unless due consideration is given to timing and siting of the thermometer in temperature recordings.

Closs (1987) describes a worrying study which showed that in a series of 43 readings taken on postoperative patients within 4.5 hours of surgery, values ranged from 0.9°C below to 1.4°C above actual temperature as measured with a highly accurate zero-gradient aural thermometer (Sloan and Keatinge, 1975).

In summarizing the mass of research evidence, Closs concludes that there is great scope for error besides inappropriate timing. However, if factors such as accurate placement of thermometer, a firmly closed mouth, and absence of hot or cold drinks in the 15–30 minutes before observation can be relied on, then 4 minutes should give a clinically significant reading. The difference between 4 and 8 minutes is only likely to be of the order of 0.2°C, which is not significant in terms of diagnosis and which, compared with other sources of error, makes the justification of an extra 4 minutes untenable.

Recommendations for good practice

1. If temperature recordings are required only daily, they should be taken between 1700 and 1900 hours. The exact time should be flexible to fit in best with the patient's activity at that time of day.
2. The thermometer should be placed in the left or right sublingual pocket, and the recording should be taken with the patient's mouth closed. The thermometer should be in place for 4 minutes.

'Her blood pressure is 147 over 96, Sister.'

Blood pressure readings are an important screening tool. Serial measurements are essential to monitor the patient's cardiovascular status in critical situations, postoperatively and in cases of cardiovascular disease.

Once again this task is usually assigned to junior students, and given the complexity of what is involved, there is considerable scope for error, making comments such as the one quoted above meaningless. It is simply not possible to measure a blood pressure that accurately, as the standard for manometer accuracy is ± 3 mmHg, even if all else is perfect. In other words, at best the reading is only within 3 mmHg of the true value.

Draper (1987) has described a series of investigations showing serious inaccuracies in sphygmomanometers due to inadequate maintenance. Staff should ask themselves when the sphygmomanometers on their units were last overhauled and more crucially, how they would recognize faults in their equipment which might be leading to false readings, e.g. perished rubber tubing or a faulty valve. Cuffs are also a source of error; if they are too large for the patient they give false low readings and vice versa if too small. Draper, for example, describes an observed series of 200 blood pressure readings; in 65 of them, the cuff was incorrectly applied.

The use of automatic blood pressure recording machines has widened in the last few years. Whilst there is no published research on how well such machines are used, anecdotal evidence exists to suggest that some nurses fail to understand how to use them correctly, with the result that spurious recordings are possible. This is particularly worrying in view of the fact that patients on continuous monitoring tend to be in an unstable haemodynamic condition and errors could therefore have serious consequences.

Simple alterations in arm position introduce significant variations in readings. Webb (1980) describes how only a small raising or lowering of the arm away from the level of the heart can lower or raise blood pressure by 5 to 6 mmHg respectively. If the patient's arm is unsupported, the isometric muscular contraction needed to maintain its position raises systolic blood pressure by 8 mmHg, while the relaxing effect of supporting the patient's back can lower both systolic and diastolic blood pressure by 8 mmHg.

Even the choice of arm can affect blood pressure. A study by Kristensen (1982) found that in a sample of 197 men and women, 49% had differences in systolic blood pressure of greater than 10 mmHg between arms. Similar discrepancies in diastolic blood pressure occurred in 29% of the sample.

Various sources of error are possible within the observer, such as hearing acuity, effects of environmental noise, or whether the observer chooses the muffling of sounds or the total disappearance of sounds as the diastolic pressure (phases IV and V Korotkoff sounds). This latter point is the source of much difference of opinion and clearly if different observers use different criteria for diastolic blood pressure, then different values will ensue.

It remains for us to consider the frequency with which blood pressure observations are carried out. It is again the authors' experience that the majority of patients on wards are seen to have multiple blood pressure observations daily. Two consistently parallel rows of arrows march across the observation chart, indicating a stable blood pressure. In fact, sometimes it is just too stable in view of the factors discussed above – so much so that one starts to wonder whether the blood pressure was recorded at all, or to what extent the recorded value was determined by the preceding value?

A moment's thought would indicate that on an average 30-bed ward, if two-thirds of the patients were on frequent blood pressure readings, some 2–3 nursing hours will be spent recording blood pressure each day. The reader is referred back to the discussion of temperature recording for further consideration of this excessive frequency of observation and possible waste of nursing time.

Recommendations for good practice

1. Frequency of blood pressure monitoring should be reviewed daily for each patient by a qualified nurse.
2. Recording techniques should be monitored to ensure accuracy.
3. Completed charts should be monitored as part of a quality control programme.
4. Equipment should be checked and overhauled frequently.
5. Readings should be recorded to the nearest 5 mmHg.
6. All staff should use the same definition of diastolic blood pressure.

'Mr Harrison's blood pressure is 160 over 90 and his pulse 100. Why wasn't I told of this, Staff?'
Taking a pulse is a very simple observation, yet it can give vital information about the patient's condition. However, it is possible to find that observations clearly departing from the normal have been unreported to senior staff. Is this because the junior staff who took the pulse did not realize there was a deviation from the norm or – such is the system of nursing on the ward – that there is no direct communication with a trained member of staff to whom such a reading can be reported? An alternative explanation is that such channels exist, but students are

afraid to use them because they perceive that members of the trained staff are likely to ignore them or be rude to them. Such unhealthy attitudes are major barriers to communication and unfortunately still linger in some of our hospitals today.

Pulse-taking which is part of a task-oriented approach will inevitably become a ritual and vital clues about a patient's condition may be missed. Telling a nurse to record up to 15 patients' pulses in succession on an 'obs round' is no way to give individualized care. If a nurse has a small group of patients, she or he must be encouraged to see the pulse observation as part of the whole patient. How does the pulse fit in with the other vital signs? How is it varying over time? Is there a trend? Is the pulse regular or, if irregular, in what way? How does the patient appear? How does he or she feel? Questions such as these should be in a nurse's mind when checking a pulse.

Mr Harrison, referred to at the start of this section, is likely to be anxious and worried if such elevated pulse and blood pressure readings have been recorded. Perhaps he has just been admitted as an emergency and does not understand what is happening. Maybe pain is adding to his stress. The nurse must ask if all is well and give him the opportunity to talk. Repeating the observations after such an exercise, maybe half an hour later, will probably show vital signs much nearer the norm, as his anxiety will have lessened.

'It is remarkable that every patient on this ward has a respiratory rate of 20!'

More than one consultant has been heard to make this remark on a ward round, and it would indeed be remarkable given that the normal resting respiratory rate is between 12 and 16 breaths per minute. Respiratory rate is another vital sign, and one that is most dreadfully neglected, as if nurses think it is of no importance. Wards can be visited where respiratory rate is not even recorded at all, or where a straight line through the improbably rapid rate of 20 breaths per minute min tells a story of nursing assessment that is less than expert.

Changes in rate are early signs of a host of serious conditions, varying from the obvious such as a chest infection or heart failure, to the less obvious such as fat embolism. It is not just a matter of rate. Consider also whether the rhythm is regular or irregular. Signs such as laboured breathing involving the use of the accessory muscles indicate severe respiratory distress, while shallow breathing indicates pain on inspiration. Is the shape of the chest normal? Does the chest wall expand equally on both sides? Questions such as these can be answered in seconds by just looking at the patient before checking the actual rate of breathing. Nursing observations of variables such as these are essential on admission to establish a good baseline from which to work. How is the nurse to know if a patient's breathing has become more rapid and laboured since this morning if no documented observations were carried out?

It is a fact of life that doctors may not see their patients from one day to the next. Therefore the early detection of complications such as a chest infection or pulmonary embolism is the responsibility of the nurse. Unless respiratory observations are carried out correctly on all patients, vital early signs of such complications will be missed, to the patient's cost.

If we are to avoid ritualistic practice which may be harmful to the patient, nurses must be taught the significance of observations such as respiratory rate and they must operate in a ward environment where senior staff are also aware of such factors and where staff are made responsible for the total individual care of their patients. Educationalists are responsible for the former, sisters and charge nurses the latter.

Recommendations for good practice

1. Pulse and respiratory rate and rhythm should be recorded daily, or more frequently if the patient's condition indicates.
2. Frequency of observation should be reviewed daily by the qualified nurse who is responsible for the patient.
3. Other signs associated with respiration should also be monitored if appropriate, e.g. depth of breathing, pain associated with breathing.

Nurses now measure more patient variables than the basic four vital signs. Diabetic patients have always had their urine tested for glucose and modern practice sees nurses carrying out the more accurate and clinically relevant monitoring of blood glucose levels using one of the commercially available reagent strip methods – capillary blood glucose monitoring or CBGM, as it is known. The question must be asked whether nurses fully understand the theory of what they are doing. Has this task become based on an incorrect understanding of theory, upon mythology, or has it become just another daily chore?

A study by Almond (1986) has raised the alarm that this may indeed be the case. Anecdotal evidence quoted in her paper reveals nurses using urine-testing strips to test blood; nurses recording readings of 4 mmol/litre when a lab test on venous blood was 94 mmol/litre or, conversely, a patient given insulin because of a high reagent stick reading while the lab result was only 3.4 mmol/litre. Almond is able to quote research demonstrating that the basic technique is reliable, especially with the use of a meter, providing the readings are carried out in compliance with the manufacturer's instructions. As is often the case, there is nothing wrong with the instrument; it is how humans use it that causes errors.

Self-administered CBGM greatly improves the quality of care for diabetic patients at home and is an essential part of their inpatient management. If the patient is expected to perform the measurement accurately, the nurse should also be capable of reaching the same standard.

In her study Almond visited 30 wards and observed 35 CBGM readings; 26 used a meter and 9 were done with the naked eye. After each nurse reading, the researcher obtained a specimen of capillary blood from the subject and sent it for laboratory examination.

For purposes of clinical practice, CBGM is acceptable if readings are within 20% of a path lab determination. Of 21 readings done with a Glucometer, 11 failed this criterion while 1 in 4 of the readings made with a Hypocount 2B meter was also unacceptable. Of the naked-eye readings, 5 out of 9 were unacceptable.

These results represent only one reading on each ward, but are a major cause for concern and indicate the need for an urgent replication of this study on a larger scale. The reasons behind over 50% of these results being more than 20% in error were not hard to find. Almond lists a worrying series of mistakes made by the nurses carrying out the procedures and describes dirty equipment and the use of test sticks over a year out of date in one case. The grades of staff making such vital observations ranged from unqualified nursing auxiliaries to ward sisters.

The reality of nursing practice as revealed by this research is a depressing one. A simple yet vital observation, essential for the safe management and care of a common yet potentially fatal illness, lies beyond the scope of over half the nurses in this study. In seeking to explain these poor nursing standards, the quality of teaching given to the nurses must come in for close scrutiny. Nurse teachers have a case to answer if their methods still smack of rote-learning. Such an approach leads to nurses learning only what to do, without learning the theory behind it. The lack of a theoretical base for nursing action predisposes to ritual, and in this case may explain the less than satisfactory standard of observations. The quality of these measurements clearly has implications for the standards of care afforded to such diabetic patients.

Recommendations for good practice

1. CGBM should be carried out strictly in accordance with the manufacturer's instructions.
2. Ward sisters or charge nurses should update their own knowledge and check the performance of their staff.
3. A small-scale quality control exercise, as described above, should be implemented as an on-going exercise in each hospital.
4. New techniques should only be introduced after a proper in-service training programme has been carried out.

'We need half-hourly abdominal girth measurements on Mr McClean, Nurse.'

Abdominal girth measurements have traditionally been carried out to detect intra-abdominal bleeding, the rationale being that a collection of fluid (blood) within the abdominal cavity will be revealed by an increase in abdominal girth.

There are two major problems with this belief, which research has shown is a dangerous myth. Firstly there are problems with the accuracy of measurements. Secondly, the quantity of free blood required to produce measurable changes would be so great that the clinical signs of shock would have been apparent some time earlier.

To obtain accurate readings the observer must apply exactly the same amount of tension on the tape measure each time a reading is taken. This is unlikely to happen, and when different observers are used the reliability of the observations is questionable. (We are all familiar with how easy it is to deceive oneself that a size 12 skirt will still fit by tightening the tape measure a little!) Other problems relate to the possibility of readings being taken in different positions on the abdomen and the tendency of observers to repeat the observation of their predecessor and get the same result. What is expected tends to be what is found.

Fairclough et al (1984) investigated the accuracy of readings by asking a group of 10 qualified nurses and junior doctors to measure a subject's abdominal girth 10 times each, over a 2.5 hour period. The subject was a 26-year-old male lying in bed; he had emptied his bladder just before the experiment began. One further refinement was to remove lengths of between 1 and 5 cm from the linen tape used. This simulated increases in abdominal girth of those amounts.

The results were that, with the tape of constant length, there was a range of 6 cm in the readings made on the same abdomen; 8 of the 10 observers failed to detect an apparent increase of 3 cm in girth (due to the tape being shortened by 3 cm). Some observers failed to detect any change at all, even when the tape was shortened by 5 cm.

Fairclough et al (1984) then evaluated the concept that blood loss into the abdominal cavity has to be so severe that shock would already be obvious before any increase in abdominal girth was measured. One of the research team measured the abdominal girth of 11 patients undergoing peritoneal dialysis after 1 and 2 litre exchanges. He found that the mean increase in abdominal girth was 1.65 cm/litre. The effect of losing 1–2 litres of blood is very serious; there is hypotension and all the signs of hypovolaemic shock. However, Fairclough et al's results show that most nurses (and doctors) would not recognize the 3 cm increase in abdominal girth that this loss would produce. Further, the difference between any two observers taking measurements at the same time could be 6 cm – twice the actual increase due to bleeding.

The practice of measuring abdominal girth to assess intra-abdominal blood loss was described by Fairclough et al as dangerously misleading. One can only concur with their opinion in the light of these findings. This is another myth that should be recognized as such and the practice of abdominal girth measurements should be discarded.

There are many other areas of observation and measurement that could be addressed here, including pressure sore risk, fluid balance and incontinence. These latter two points will be addressed in the next chapter on charting, while the following chapter looks at pressure sores.

References

Almond J. (1986). Measuring blood glucose levels. *Nursing Times*, **82**: 41, 51–4.

Closs J. (1987). Oral temperature measurement. *Nursing Times*, **83**: 1, 36–9.

Draper P. (1987). Not a job for juniors. *Nursing Times*, **83**: 10, 58–62.

Durham M. L., Swanson B., Paulford N. (1986). Effect of tachycardia on oral temperature estimation. *Nursing Research*, **35**, 4.

Fairclough J., Mintowt-Czyz W. J., Mackie I., Nokes L. (1984). Abdominal girth: an unreliable measure of intra-abdominal bleeding. *Injury*, **16**, 85–7.

Forster B., Adler D. C., Davis M. (1970). Duration of effects of drinking iced water on temperature. *Nursing Research*, **19**, 169–70.

Kristensen B. O. (1982). Which arm to measure blood pressure. Scand (suppl.) 69–73.

Kunnel M. T., O'Brien C., Munro B. H. (1988). Comparison of rectal, femoral, axillary and skin mattress temperatures in stable neonates. *Nursing Research*, **37**, 162–4.

Lee R. E., Atkins E. (1972). Spurious Fever. *American Journal of Nursing*, **72**,

Samples J. et al (1985). Circadian rhythms: basis for screening for fever. *Nursing Research*, **34**, 377–9.

Sloan R. E. G., Keatinge W. R. (1975). Depression of sublingual temperature by cold saliva. *British Medical Journal*, **1**, 1718–20.

Webb C. H. (1980). The measurement of blood pressure. *Primary Care*, **7**, 4.

Wintle C. (1988). A study of time taken for temperature recordings. Unpublished degree thesis, Bristol Polytechnic.

6 *Charting observations*

It is of no value for a nurse to make an observation unless it is subsequently recorded for the benefit of other staff. Such recording needs to be accurate, clear, concise and in a form that is readily available. Variables such as vital signs are not the only observations that require charting; neurological status, wound size, fluid balance, continence patterns, pain and pressure sore risk are just some examples of patient information essential for planning effective nursing care.

Reference has already been made in the previous chapter to the sort of ritualistic approach to vital sign observation that results in inaccurate measurements being charted. One further point that needs to be made concerns the various strange ways that nurses connect dots on graphs. At school, children are taught in maths that to plot a graph, points are either connected by straight lines or smooth curves depending on the nature of the mathematical functions involved. They are also taught that a graph begins at the beginning with the first observation made.

A glance at many of the charts hanging from bed ends shows that these simple rules of maths have been superseded by some strange hospital rituals that result in graphs being positively misleading. Figure 1 contains some examples. Nurses should follow the basic rules of drawing graphs learnt at school if the charts they produce are to be accurate and give a true impression of the patient's progress (Figure 2).

'Miss Webb is drowsy and a bit confused today, Sister.'
What exactly does this statement mean? It is very subjective – what is drowsy to one nurse may not be drowsy to another – and is Miss Webb confused in time or space, or has she just forgotten where she put her knitting? Nurses need to try and quantify in an objective way their assessment of a patient's neurological status, whether the patient is an acute head injury or recovering from a stroke. The Glasgow coma scale (Walsh, 1985) should be used for this purpose as it provides objective measurements of a patient's level of consciousness.

If neurological observation is to make sense then the same nurse should make the observations on a patient for the duration of her shift;

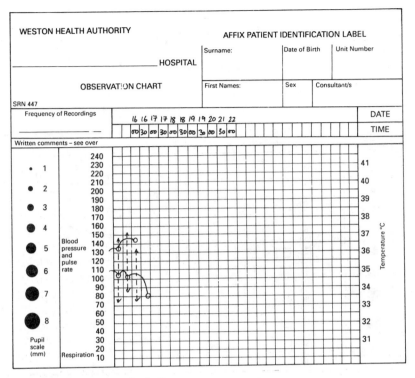

Figure 1 *Common errors in charting*

1 *No name or identification*
2 *Frequency of recordings not written in*
3 *No times recorded for first two sets of observations*
4 *It is not clear which line refers to temperature and which to pulse*
5 *Individual temperature and pulse observations are not accurately marked; circles rather than points or crosses have been used*
6 *Point values are not joined by straight lines*
7 *No respiratory observations have been carried out*
8 *It is assumed that observations will be carried out half-hourly until 2200 hours; changes in the patient's condition may cause observations to be carried out more or less frequently*

in this way, observed changes are more likely to be real changes rather than apparent ones caused by different personnel making the observations.

Nurses should ask why they are carrying out neurological observations on a patient if their care is to avoid becoming ritualistic. Consider the practice of observing pupil size. This is done to detect the effects of an expanding intracranial lesion compressing the third cranial nerve, usually

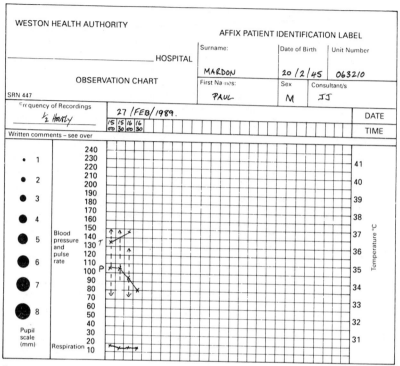

Figure 2   *The same observations correctly chartered*

in the case of trauma. If the patient has taken an overdose of drugs, pupil size will simply be determined by the drugs taken and will have no relation to any intracerebral pathology, so why observe their size? If the patient is awake, alert and oriented after head injury, there cannot be an expanding lesion compressing the third cranial nerve as this will have long ago produced a reduction in level of consciousness, so why check the patient's pupils, blood pressure and pulse every half hour? Decreased level of consciousness is the first sign of head injury, apparent before any of the other signs that are ritualistically monitored every half-hour.

How else except by ritual can we explain the following situation? A patient returned from theatre after having a lacerated nerve in his hand repaired. The nurse was asked to carry out neurological observations, so she faithfully checked the patient's pupil size, blood pressure and pulse every half-hour, but never the sensation or movement in the patient's hand which was, of course, the whole point of the exercise.

Consider the nurse in the Accident & Emergency department caring for a child who had suffered a fracture dislocation of the elbow. This injury carries a major risk of serious neurovascular damage affecting the forearm if the brachial artery and/or a nerve (e.g. ulnar nerve) becomes trapped in the disrupted joint. The nurse was asked to check the child's pulse every 15 minutes (to ensure a patent blood supply to the forearm), so she neatly recorded the pulse rate on a chart and quickly told the charge nurse checking the child's circulation that the pulse was 90 and she was being careful to take it in the *uninjured* arm in order to avoid hurting the child! Fortunately this child did not develop a Volkmann's ischaemic contracture as her brachial artery escaped damage.

Examples such as these lead one to conclude that some nurses learn a standard reflex response to the phrase 'neurological observations' and carry out a task-centred ritual without due regard to the individual patient's condition, resulting in wasted time and effort and, possibly, hazard to the patient.

Recommendations for good practice

1. Neurological observations should be appropriate to the condition of the patient and should be carried out by the same nurse for the duration of her shift.
2. Charting should be clear and accurate.

'I don't know if Mrs Donvan's leg ulcer is any better because I haven't dressed it before.'

The progress of wound healing needs to be monitored if the effectiveness of dressing techniques is to be evaluated. The chances are that several different nurses will dress the same wound in a short space of time – though primary nursing should reduce the numbers involved – therefore the only way a nurse can know if progress is being made is by accurate charting of wound size and appearance or by the use of photographs taken at regular intervals. This applies equally to a burn or leg ulcer being dressed on an outpatient basis in Accident & Emergency or the community as it does to a pressure sore on a ward patient.

We have seen in previous chapters that a mass of myth surrounds the subject of wound dressings. Repeated dressings without careful evaluation of their effectiveness is another example of unthinking ritual practice.

One simple method of monitoring healing is to make a sketch of the wound with the dimensions marked in, giving a description of its appearance, and a note about the type of dressing used. This information however needs standardizing as, for example, one nurse may remark on whether there is an odour, while another may not.

Cuzzell (1986) offers one such approach with two different checklists that can be used with either a closed or open wound. Thus in checking a closed wound the presence or absence of features such as localized tenderness, purulent drainage or erythema of the suture line may be indicated by ticking in the appropriate column as either present or absent. Features of an open wound such as odour, adherent necrotic tissue and tenderness at the margins may be recorded in the same way. Combining such a wound assessment flowsheet with simple sketches can give the nursing staff caring for the patient invaluable information about the healing process, and also provide a database for research into the effectiveness of different dressing techniques.

Accurate charting has one further advantage in relation to medical staff ward rounds. If the ward staff are able to produce accurate information on wound healing, it is no longer necessary for the dressing to be removed for inspection several times a week. Such repeated and unnecessary procedures increase the risk of introducing infection and delay healing by disturbing newly formed tissue, drying the wound out and reducing its temperature as a result of exposure.

Accurate and regular wound charting represents a movement away from ritualistic to rational care. The small amount of extra time spent on such charting will be saved many times over by ensuring more effective treatment of the patient and a shorter healing time. There are also significant financial savings to be made, as we saw previously.

'It's funny, only four patients have IVIs at the moment, but nearly everybody seems to be on a fluid balance chart.'
Many patients in hospital, regardless of age or medical problems, are prone to dehydration or problems with passing urine. Accurate measurement of fluid intake and output is therefore essential. In normal health we take care of this aspect of physiology automatically. However in illness this is not so. A survey by Turner and Turner (1987) revealed that of 927 hospital patients, 36% were unable to drink independently. This suggests that about one-third of hospital patients require careful monitoring of their fluid balance and assistance with fluid intake, whether orally or parenterally, if dehydration is to be avoided.

It is a common experience however to walk on to wards and find nearly every patient is on a fluid balance chart, including patients who are ambulant, able to drink normally and void urine without a catheter. The explanation again is to be found in nurses ritualistically doing what they have always done without thinking or asking questions. 'If he was on a fluid chart yesterday then he should be on one today' is the logic. Or is it a case of the nurse having no immediately valid reason for having a patient on a fluid balance chart, but doing it 'just in case'? It could be argued that nurses do many things that are unnecessary 'just in case'. This seems to indicate a lack of confidence in their clinical judgement, perhaps because nurses are not used to being free to make decisions on care. Rather they have been trained to do what they are told by senior persons in authority, usually doctors. Recent developments such as individualized care have put nurses in the position of having to make and be accountable for their own decisions. Many nurses seem uneasy with this responsibility and so tend to do things which they know are not necessary, just in case someone in authority asks why something was not done. To many nurses it is easier to carry out a mass of unnecessary observations so that something may be produced, just in case such a question is asked, rather than defend a clinical judgement that this observation was not needed.

In the same way that patients may be on unnecessary observations, so too some patients are on fluid balance charts unnecessarily. Thinking nursing and individualized nursing should prevent the ritual of all patients being on fluid balance charts.

When so many patients are on charts, the reliability of those charts starts to become open to question. How accurately are they filled in? Our guess is that in such situations the answer is 'not very'. It is possible to look at charts and find no entry has been made for 6 hours. Nurses come round at lunchtime or even early afternoon asking patients what they had to drink that morning. How reliable is the patient's memory? A standard National Health Service cup appears to be made of elastic as it can hold 150 ml of tea in one health authority and 180 ml in another. The quantity drunk is not recorded, only the quantity dispensed. How many untouched cold cups of tea go down the drain and down on the fluid balance chart as having been drunk?

Another common ritual is the 1 litre water jug. This is put out on the patient's locker by the domestic staff in the morning. It is assumed that any fluid not in this jug at 2100 hours has been drunk by the patient and thus is entered on the fluid balance chart. What justification is there for this assumption? Absolutely none – water could be spilt, poured on flowers, given to another patient or poured out and forgotten about, to name but four possibilities. The validity of this practice should be the subject of research, as well as the patient's opinion of a jug of water that has been standing in a warm environment for 12 hours as a suitably appealing drink.

The present system of charting oral fluid intake is often ritualistic and may bear little resemblance to the true situation, as it is assumed that all that is presented to the patient is drunk by the patient. Nursing care plans mentioning 'pushing fluids' make one wonder if any progress has been made in the last 15 years towards nursing care that is individualized and based on measurable patient-centred goals. Turner and Turner (1988) point out that a fluid intake of less than 1200 ml/day requires supplementation to prevent dehydration. Given the suspected poor standards of fluid balance monitoring that may exist in some areas, it may be asked how many patients have fallen below this limit without nursing staff being aware?

Recommendations for good practice

1. Patients on fluid balance charts should be reviewed daily to see if they can be discontinued.

2. A small number of essential and accurate charts is better than a large number of unnecessary charts that are incorrectly filled in.

3. Fluid drunk should be recorded, not fluid offered.

'Miss Nolan is wet again, Sister. I don't know how many times that is today.'

A logical step from fluid intake is to look at output, and in particular to consider the problem of incontinence. Moody (1989) has explored many of the myths and rituals surrounding incontinence, especially the myth that it is somehow an inevitable aspect of ageing and nothing can be done about it. Nothing could be further from the truth, of course.

There are many interventions that can either eliminate the problem or greatly relieve the effects on the patient. Like all nursing, care must start with assessment and as Rooney (1987) has pointed out, a toileting chart will identify the baseline of the problem and can act as a great aid to continence. Rooney considers that it is impossible for staff to give an accurate description verbally of how often any one patient is incontinent, reminding the nurse to try and recall exactly when and how many times she herself has been to the toilet in the last 24 hours. Charting is therefore necessary.

Various charts are available, depending on the needs of the patient. Some are designed to be filled in by both nurse and patient, others by nurse alone. The result should be an accurate picture of the patient's continence upon which to base a logical plan of care aimed at restoring full continence and dispelling the myth of once incontinent, always incontinent. If the chart shows frequency, urinary tract infection or anxiety may be causative factors; dribbling suggests overflow incontinence and retention while night wetness may indicate excess sedation or difficulty in getting assistance with toileting. Not only can progress be monitored but vital information can be gained into possible causes of the patient's continence problems. Continence charting is a good example of rational nursing care that will help to dispel some of the myths surrounding this problem.

References

Cuzzell J. Z. (1986). Tell it like it is. *American Journal of Nursing*, **86**, 600–1.

Moody, M. (1989). *Incontinence*. Heinemann: Oxford.

Rooney V. (1987). Toileting charts. *Nursing*, **3**, 827–30.

Turner A., Turner J. (1987). Problems of recognizing dehydration in hospital patients. *Nursing Times*, **83**: 51, 49.

Turner A., Turner J. (1988). Helping the dehydrated patient. *Nursing Times*, **84**: 18, 40–1.

Walsh M. (1985). *A&E Nursing, A New Approach*. Heinemann: Oxford.

7 Pressure sores

Pressure sores are a well recognized serious complication of any condition associated with immobility. They are also largely preventable, though the increasing numbers of elderly debilitated patients who survive for lengthy periods present a major challenge to nursing in the field of pressure sore prevention. Unfortunately this field remains the subject of a mass of nursing folklore and while many areas approach the problem from a rational base with good results, there are also many other practising nurses locked into ritualistic patterns of care based on fiction not fact.

In order to sift out fact from fiction, rituals from rational action, a basic understanding of the cause of pressure sores is required. Versluysen (1986) analyses causative factors into two groups — intrinsic and extrinsic. Extrinsic factors consist of shearing forces within the tissue planes and localized pressure over bony prominences exceeding capillary pressure (28–38 mmHg), leading to occlusion of the microcirculation and tissue necrosis. It has been shown that the duration of excess pressure rather than the amount of pressure is the most important factor in tissue necrosis. Thus a pressure of 100 mmHg applied for 2 hours will cause as much damage as a pressure of 600 mmHg applied for 1 hour (Exton-Smith, 1987).

Intrinsic factors are concerned with the patient rather than the forces acting on the patient's skin and include age, incontinence, physique, other concurrent disease, nutritional status and the presence of infection.

In order to come to grips with this huge area, the rest of this chapter will consider the extent of the problem, measures for prevention and the treatment of established sores. It is hoped that by stripping away some of the mythology, a more rational approach to care will be developed.

'We don't have pressure sores on this ward.'
Gould (1985) described an interesting guilt phenomenon amongst nurses which emerged during research into their knowledge of pressure care. Some nurses felt that no patient should ever develop a sore, therefore

they felt guilty when some did. Could this guilt lead to denial and the sort of statement quoted above?

Nyquist and Hawthorn (1987) undertook a major study of a large health authority (Nottingham) to determine the incidence of pressure sores in all hospital inpatients, with the exceptions of acute psychiatry and obstetrics. The authors are able to quote work showing that nurses in a previous study documented only 73% of existing pressure sores (poor observation, poor recording or denial and guilt?) and therefore point out that their figures are probably an underestimate of the incidence.

The study looked at a total of 2513 patients in 133 wards and revealed that 132 patients had 233 documented pressure sores. This gives a rate of 5.3% across the authority; highest figures were on the care of the elderly wards (10.7%) and orthopaedic wards (9.3%). Of the 132 with pressure sores, 80.3% were aged over 65. Another way of looking at this figure is to say that 47% of the patients with sores were on care of the elderly wards; the survey also revealed that these wards had the lowest staffing levels of all wards in the health authority.

Amongst the patients' medical conditions, 32 had arthritis or rheumatoid disease, 31 had disease of the cardiovascular system, 22 were suffering paralysis after a stroke and 20 had malignant disease. A total of 22 of the 132 were reported as suffering from dementia.

The distribution of sores revealed that the most common site was the buttocks or sacral area (54.9% of all sores) followed by the foot and ankle area (24.9%). The worst sores in terms of area and depth were located in the buttocks or sacral region.

'The only patients with pressure sores on this ward come in with them.'

This rationalization offers an easy escape from guilt feelings. Unfortunately there is substantial evidence to show that many patients develop their sores in hospital. Versluysen (1985) demonstrated that 66% of patients admitted with fractures involving the hip developed pressure sores in hospital. Of this group, 83% developed their sores within 5 days of admission.

This particular medical condition occurs almost exclusively amongst the elderly and involves immobilization for at least 24 hours, although the whole thrust of orthopaedic surgery is to aim for the earliest possible mobilization. Areas such as Accident & Emergency, the X-ray department and theatres are all implicated in the causation of pressure sores as trolleys in these areas have been shown to generate pressures well in excess of the capillary pressure needed to maintain tissue perfusion (Versluysen, 1986). Lengthy stays of several hours in Accident & Emergency are commonplace for such patients, and tissue breakdown will probably have started before the patient even gets to the orthopaedic ward. Accident & Emergency units and operating theatres need to implement pressure area care as well as wards.

Warner and Hall (1986) investigated the development of pressure sores after admission in a 4-week study of a large general hospital, involving 396 patients. They found that no orthopaedic or surgical admissions had pressure sores, but that 28% of admissions to the elderly care unit did. Significantly, of 334 patients admitted without sores, 26 developed them.

Exton-Smith (1987) has looked closely at the incidence of pressure sores in a large specialized care of the elderly unit. He found an overall incidence of 24% amongst a series of 250 patients. He was also able to show that 70% of the sores which developed in the unit did so in the first 2 weeks and that patients over 85 developed sores at twice the rate as did those under 75.

The evidence demonstrates that, while some patients come into hospital with pressure sores, particularly the elderly, many sores develop while in hospital and tend to do so in the first 2 weeks of hospitalization. Nurses have to be honest and admit that patients do develop pressure sores on wards. It is a myth to say otherwise.

'All patients on this ward get the pressure area care they need.'

A statement such as this invites some questions. Firstly, do all the patients need pressure care, and if not, how does the nurse decide which patients need care and which do not? If time is being spent on some patients who do not need pressure area care, this suggests that time could be better spent on others who really do need intensive pressure area care. Could this help to explain why patients continue to develop pressure sores despite protestations that all patients receive the care they need? The root of the problem lies in the methods used to assess which patients need pressure area care.

In addition we need to consider whether nurses actually give the care they say they do and finally, are nurses using correct methods that have been demonstrated to work, or is clinical practice dominated by outdated ideas and beliefs which are all part of the mythology of nursing?

A routinized, ritualistic approach to pressure care leads to the sort of blanket assertion made above – that all patients receive pressure care.

Yet somehow pressure sores keep on developing. Many patients do not need pressure care, they are mobile and can therefore take care of their pressure areas for themselves. What is needed is some sort of assessment tool that will discriminate, that will allow nurses to pick out those patients most at risk of pressure area problems, so that the limited nursing resources available can be concentrated on these patients. Many nurses say they rely on 'professional judgement' when asked how they would assess at-risk patients. At best this is a rather nebulous concept and at worst little more than a subjective hunch. It is necessary to see if there is a better way of doing things.

One of the authors (Pauline Ford) has undertaken just such an exercise, having become concerned at the need to see that the limited amount of nursing time available on her unit was deployed to the best effect. A decision was taken to review the criteria used to decide which patients on this care of the elderly unit needed pressure area care. The previous system of leaving it to the subjective professional judgement of the nurse was replaced with the objective scoring system for assessing risk developed by Norton et al (1962). The result was a major improvement; pressure area care was given regularly and correctly to those who demonstrably needed it.

It is now over a quarter of a century since Norton et al (1962) gave nursing the tool it needs for pressure area risk assessment yet many areas still do not use it as part of their nursing assessment. Norton et al advocated scoring patients from 1 to 4 on five different dimensions – physical condition, mental state, activity, mobility and incontinence. A patient could therefore score a top mark of 20, providing he or she was fully alert, ambulant, mobile, continent and in good physical condition. Norton et al's research indicated that if patients scored 14 or less they were at high risk of developing pressure sores.

One myth that has grown up in nursing is that if the patient scored over 14 he or she is at no risk. This is not so, and this was never stated by the authors. Norton et al affirmed that patients were at less risk, but that some element of risk remained. It is up to the nurse to take other factors into account in making a judgement about patients scoring over 14.

Barratt (1987) has discussed the value of the Norton system and other comparable methods. Criticisms levelled at the Norton scale include the fact that it was developed only for use with the elderly, it takes no account of patient pathology, nutritional status or pain, and that it is rather crude. Pajk et al (1987) have investigated the problem and felt that the most common problem encountered in patients with pressure sores was impaired nutritional status, followed by impaired activity and mobility, then incontinence and finally impaired mental state. They are therefore critical of the Norton scale as it does not refer directly to nutrition. However, it must be pointed out that the general physical condition of the patient (one of Norton's five measures) is closely related to nutritional status.

Goldstone and Goldstone (1982) have criticized the Norton scale on the grounds that it overpredicts the numbers of at-risk patients, though their study was based on only a small sample. It could be argued that if a score is to have an error, it is better to err on the side of over- rather than underprediction.

Another attempt to deal with the problem is the Douglas calculator, but as Barratt (1987) points out, there has been no validation of this system. Even Goldstone and Goldstone (1982), despite their criticisms, were forced to acknowledge that the Norton system remains a reliable guide to those patients most at risk.

It is interesting to return to the studies on pressure sore frequency described above and see how the Norton scale fared. In the Nottingham series (Nyquist and Hawthorn, 1987), 91 patients with pressure sores scored 14 or less (61.9%); however, it should be noted that 11 patients classed as ambulant or fully mobile did develop pressure sores. Exton-Smith's (1987) study revealed that 48% of patients with sores scored less than 12, but 5% of patients with sores scored 18–20. From a slightly different point of view, Warner and Hall's figures allowed them to identify 51 patients who had been hospitalized for over 2 weeks with a Norton score of 14 or less; 17 of these (33%) developed pressure sores.

The conclusion drawn from these three studies of hospital populations is that the Norton system is very effective in predicting pressure sore development. In the last study for example, a third of patients identified developed pressure sores, *despite active nursing care*. The fact that the Norton scale was devised after a study of elderly patients suggests that its predictive value will however be best when applied to such patients.

Warner and Hall point out that the group of patients aged over 65 who scored 14 or less and who spent at least 2 weeks in hospital accounted for 58% of all cases of pressure sores that developed in the 4-week period of their study. The fact that this group numbered only 43 of a total of 396 patients in the whole study indicates how effective the Norton scale can be in picking out very high-risk patients.

A simple, reliable tool is therefore available to nurses to identify high-risk patients. It is a myth to say that it is impossible to predict who will develop pressure sores. It is a myth to say that the Norton scale does not work. Attempts at carrying out pressure care on all patients becomes a ritual which is harmful to those who most need it as there is not the time to give them the full care they need. Those units using the Norton scale are basing their care on rational assessment; areas that do not seem to be relying on subjective intuition. Many surgical, orthopaedic and medical wards and Accident & Emergency units are prime examples of areas which should be using this scale, but which one suspects are not.

'Rubbing the skin with meths prevents pressure sores.'

Here is just one myth among many in the field of pressure sore prevention. Experience suggests it is still practised and research by Anthony (1987) confirms this is so. The use of oils or meths will promote skin breakdown and destroy normal skin flora and fats, paving the way for skin necrosis and infection.

There is no evidence to show that the use of barrier creams and talcum powder reduces the incidence of pressure sores, although they may seriously interfere with the normal functions of skin. No agent applied to the skin has been demonstrated to reduce the incidence of pressure sores. Such ritualistic practices therefore are of no demonstrated value and may be of real harm.

Consideration of the basic causes of pressure sores should lead to the simple conclusion that the best way to prevent them is to prevent pressure and shearing frictional forces upon the skin. This is the single most effective method. Exton-Smith (1987) has described a study in which a rigorous 2-hourly turning regime was introduced for at-risk patients in a unit where early pressure sore development was running at 19%. The effect was a reduction in a sample of 100 patients to an incidence of 4%.

In view of this finding, the 2-hourly turning regime is confirmed as the rational basis for preventing pressure sores. The findings of Gould (1985) are therefore somewhat disturbing. She discovered many areas of inadequate knowledge amongst nurses about pressure sores and was particularly alarmed to find that, in her sample of nurses, 16.3% thought that the use of a pressure-preventing aid made it unnecessary to turn the patient. Another myth, another pressure sore.

What then is the value of a ripple bed or a sheepskin? A wide range of ripple beds are available, but many suffer from the problem that they are only effective if the patient is lying flat. Sitting the patient at, say, 45° imposes a major shearing stress over the sacral area proportional to the weight of the whole upper part of the body.

Exton-Smith therefore recommends the Pegasus Airwave system as the best choice because it is possible to sit a patient up to 60°, yet the portion of the cycle that generates maximum pressure over the sacrum is less than 20% of the whole, which should be within the limits of what the tissues in that area can tolerate. The Mediscus Low Air Loss Bed is also considered capable of providing protection from shearing forces over the sacrum.

The use of a ripple mattress alone will not prevent pressure sores – that is a myth. Sitting a patient up while on a ripple mattress largely invalidates the beneficial effects of the mattress, unless it is one of the two systems described above.

A frequently encountered aid to prevent pressure sores is the sheepskin, designed to prevent friction, thereby reducing shearing forces on the tissues beneath the skin. However, a sheepskin does not reduce the pressure directly on the skin, therefore sitting a patient or resting a limb on a sheepskin will not reduce the need for turning to relieve that pressure. The pressure must be relieved every 2 hours; the sheepskin merely reduces friction during movement. It is not uncommon to find sheepskins used incorrectly, as though they relieve direct pressure in some mysterious way.

If friction and shearing forces are major contributory factors in the aetiology of pressure sores then it is a reasonable hypothesis that the occlusive film-type dressings which greatly reduce friction might be effective in preventing pressure sores (e.g. OpSite, Tegaderm). Anecdotal evidence is available to suggest that they do have a beneficial effect in preventing the breakdown of vulnerable areas. A carefully controlled investigation into how effective such dressings might be in the prophylaxis of pressure sores would therefore be a worthwhile project.

It is a fact that this type of dressing meets many of the criteria for wound care. It would be a great bonus if they could be shown to prevent pressure sores as well as being an effective treatment of established sores.

An essential step for patients in mobilization and recovery is that they should sit out of bed as soon as possible. However, once there, some nurses seem to forget about their pressure care and they are left sitting for 3–6 hours in the same position with no relief of pressure over their buttocks. In some way, sitting out of bed seems to be all that is needed.

If the patient is stood up every 1–2 hours, encouraged to take a few steps or offered assistance in getting to the toilet, there will be many other benefits in terms of mobility and rehabilitation, apart from the obvious benefit of pressure relief over the buttocks and sacrum.

An observant eye will note that, when sat out of bed, the patient's feet are often put up on a footstool, ensuring that there is maximum pressure over the heel – pressure that remains unbroken (unlike the patient's skin) for several hours. If the rationale for this action is to assist venous return, then to be effective the legs must be elevated far higher than they are in practice, ideally above the level of the heart. If feet must be put on a footstool, a little thought would indicate the need to arrange pillows in such a way as to keep the heel free from pressure.

The nurse should be aware that the natural position of comfort for the knee is slightly flexed at about 10°. Keeping the leg straight while sat out of bed is therefore putting the knee joint in an unnatural and uncomfortable position. Thought should also be given to the position of the patient's hip and whole body posture while sat out of bed, particuarly if the individual is elderly, arthritic or unable to change position due to a hemiplegia, for example. Closer liaison between nurses and the physiotherapy department would be beneficial to both patients and nurses.

A lot of attention is devoted to making the sacrum free from pressure when turning a patient from side to side in bed. A strange ritual occasionally witnessed by the authors involves rubbing the buttocks to 'improve the circulation'. Friction causes pressure sores. Such rituals therefore cause pressure sores, not prevent them. Despite the fact that the heels and ankles are the second most common areas for pressure sores (p. 71), it is rare for an effort to be made to relieve the pressure on these vulnerable areas. The simple insertion of a pillow under the legs will suffice to raise the heels off the bed. The patient requires *thinking* care, not *ritualistic* care.

One further device needs to be considered – the ring cushion. This may be either a rubber ring put under the patient's buttocks, or a smaller ring, often made from bandages. Lowthian (1985) has shown that while this device may relieve pressure on the area within the ring, it merely transfers the pressure to the area in contact with the cushion, causing circulatory impairment and predisposing to further tissue breakdown and oedema of the tissues within the ring. Lowthian calls for the abolition of the ring cushion as a nursing aid, a view strongly supported by the present authors. It is another traditional piece of equipment that has been shown to be more than useless – it is positively harmful.

'Sister always likes egg white and oxygen for pressure sores.'
If preventive measures have failed and the patient has developed a pressure sore or has been admitted with one in situ, the question then

arises of healing that sore as soon as possible. There seems to be a mythical belief amongst some nurses that pressure sores are in some way different from other sorts of wounds and that this justifies some of the bizarre rituals that masquerade as nursing care. If pressure sores are treated as any other wound, care should become more rational.

A major factor in delaying healing is the presence of infection. This applies in pressure sores as in any other wound, yet half the nurses in Gould's (1985) survey failed to acknowledge the fact that infection delays healing of pressure sores. A survey by David et al (1983) considered 1222 sores, reporting that infection was present in many of them, delaying healing. Clearly, infection must be eliminated before healing can be promoted.

Another popular myth uncovered by Gould (1985) was the belief that pressure sores absorb oxygen from the air, hence if nurses keep the sores open and hose them down with piped oxygen, healing is promoted. As we saw in Chapter 3, this drying effect considerably delays healing. Tissues around a pressure sore derive their oxygen supply in the same way as the rest of the body — from the blood — hence the rationale for preventing pressure sores by preventing pressure. It also follows that pressure must be kept off established sores if they are to heal. In a sample of 28 ward sisters, Gould found only 5 who said they would treat a clean pressure sore by relieving pressure.

Applying the basic principles of wound healing to pressure sores suggests that they should be cleared of dead tissue and infection, then allowed to heal in a moist, infection-free environment using a dressing with the characteristics described on pp. 29-30. During this healing stage, the area must be kept free of pressure to prevent further necrosis and to encourage a good blood supply.

In Chapter 4, correct methods of eliminating slough and infection from wounds were described, such as the use of intensive debriding agents such as Debrisan and Iodosorb. Solutions such as Eusol and paraffin were shown to be antiseptics of little value and possible harm, while topical antibiotics are a potential disaster. Other remedies, such as egg white and oxygen, insulin and oxygen, salt baths, gentian violet (all quoted by the sisters in Gould's study) are of no demonstrated value and inflict varying degrees of harm on the patient.

Once a pressure sore has been rendered clean, optimal healing will take place if one of the modern dressings described in Chapter 3 is used, providing the area is kept free from pressure. Attention should also be paid to other factors that promote healing, such as good nutrition.

As we have seen in this chapter the principles of good pressure care are simple and based on sound, valid research. There can therefore be no excuse for the wide range of bizarre, counterproductive or just plain useless treatments employed ritualistically by nurses in pressure care. In speculating why this sad state of affairs has arisen, it should be pointed out that there are also areas where the incidence of pressure sores is low due to rationally based, intensive prevention. Such units also tend to use modern treatments on patients admitted with sores or who develop sores after admission to achieve the best healing rates. With increasing numbers of very elderly, frail patients suffering multiple pathology, and also patients whose natural defence mechanisms have been impaired by immunosuppressive therapy or disease, it seems probable that there will be an increasing patient population at even greater risk of pressure sore development.

Nurses may adopt two opposite and equally invalid positions on the development of pressure sores. Firstly there is the view that all sores are preventable. Therefore the statement that a patient has developed a sore since admission implies bad nursing care, it is a confession of guilt. This leads to denial, so some nurses sweep pressure sores under the carpet. It is a topic they do not wish to discuss as it carries a threat to their self-esteem. This may explain the finding discussed earlier that only three-quarters of pressure sores are reported. This failure to face up to reality may lead to nurses looking the other way on the topic of pressure sores, which helps to explain the lack of progress and worrying lack of knowledge that appears to exist amongst nurses on this crucial topic.

The opposite point of view is that pressure sores are inevitable. This then becomes the thin end of the wedge. It is easy to rationalize the fact that a patient developed a sore because it was inevitable. This provides an excuse to cover poor nursing care. In truth, for some patients, pressure area breakdown is eventually going to be inevitable. It is almost as if they have outlived their skin and their very bodies as system by system starts to fail, but life goes on.

If nurses have carried out a good assessment, reassess to monitor progress and, despite a rational vigorous pressure area management programme sores develop, then there is nothing to feel guilty about.

One possible reason for much of the mythology and malpractice associated with pressure areas may well be the way the subject is taught. There is a general criticism that traditional nurse training has been just that, training rather than education. It has failed to produce thinking nurses, rather the result has been nurses who just do what they are told with the minimum of fuss. Such nurses will tend not to question outdated ritualistic practice because they have not been taught to; those who do quickly find themselves in trouble. The result is that in the end they either conform or, sadly, many leave nursing altogether. We will return to this theme later.

A second more specific reason may be that pressure area care is taught very early in a student's career, often in the first few weeks. While such an early introduction is necessary, the problem is that few schools of nursing then come back to the topic later when the student has a more advanced knowledge of physiology, pathology and practical experience of caring for patients. To give nurses the depth of knowledge about pressure care commensurate with its importance to patient welfare a much more intensive approach to teaching is required. It should be a topic that is returned to at various stages throughout the curriculum, expanded and added to as the student's knowledge and experience expand.

It is essential that in-service training departments update pressure care knowledge for staff in post. Writers such as Hibbs (1988) give good examples of how this may be achieved with subsequent benefits in the clinical area. Given the enormous cost of pressure sores to the National Health Service (Exton-Smith estimated £420 million in 1987 – enough to fund half of the nurses' pay award and major regrading exercise for 1988–9), it should be mandatory for every health authority to review as a matter of urgency its nursing practice in this field. Exton-Smith's estimate suggests that pressure sores cost the average health authority approximately £2 million per year; how much of that expenditure is preventable by good nursing care?

The concept of quality control is gradually gaining a foothold in the UK. A nursing audit of pressure care and its effectiveness should be an essential component of any health authority's quality control programme.

In Chapter 4 we discussed a lawsuit for malpractice brought against an American hospital by a patient who developed pressure sores on an intensive care unit. Moore (1987) has constructed a hypothetical case under English law which shows that it would be very easy for a patient to do the same in this country. To prove neglect, a patient would have to show that:

1. The nurse was under a legal duty to care for and not damage the patient.
2. A breach of that duty had occurred.
3. The patient suffered damage.

Moore argues that there are many situations where these three criteria could be demonstrated in patients who developed pressure sores after admission. How would a ward sister feel standing in court justifying the fact that her ward had not carried out a rational assessment with a tool such as the Norton scale, that there was no clearly written plan of care, that inappropriate actions had been taken to prevent pressure sore formation, and that sores were subsequently treated by methods which have been shown to be of no value or even detrimental to the patient's welfare? Given the increase in consumerism and legal activity in the health care system, such a day may not be far away.

Recommendations for good practice

1. All patients should have a Norton assessment carried out on admission and at weekly intervals thereafter.
2. Pressure sore prevention should be accomplished primarily by 2-hourly changes of position.
3. Aids should be seen as secondary preventive measures to be used in conjunction with position changes and should be administered appropriately.
4. Pressure-relieving rings should be withdrawn from use and practices such as rubbing the skin, applying oils or meths banned.
5. Established sores should be treated in line with the principles of wound management outlined in Chapters 3 and 4. Substances such as hypochlorites (e.g. Eusol) and paraffin, gentian violet, and egg white should be banned in the treatment of pressure sores along with saline baths and drying the area with piped oxygen.
6. Teaching on the subject should run throughout the student curriculum rather than being confined to the first few weeks and should be an essential part of in-service training.
7. An audit of pressure area management should be carried out on a regular basis by each health authority.

References

Anthony D. (1987). Are you in the dark? *Nursing Times*, **83**: 34, 25–30.
Barratt E. (1987). Putting risk calculators in their place. *Nursing Times*, **83**: 7, 65–70.
David J. et al (1983). An investigation of the care of patients with established pressure sores. Report of the Northwick Park nursing practice research unit.
Exton-Smith N. (1987). The patient's not for turning. *Nursing Times*, **83**: 42, 42–4.

Goldstone L. A., Goldstone J. (1982). The Norton scale: an early warning on pressure sores? *Journal of Advanced Nursing*, **7**, 419–26.

Hibbs P. (1988). Action against pressure sores. *Nursing Times*, **84**: 13, 68–73.

Gould D. (1985). Pressure for change. *Nursing Mirror*, **161**: 9, 28–30.

Lowthian P. (1985). A sore point. *Nursing Mirror*, **161**: 9, 30–3.

Moore D. (1987). The buck stops with you. *Nursing Times*, **83**: 39, 54–6.

Norton D., McLaren R., Exton-Smith A. N. (1962). *An investigation of Geriatric Nursing Problems in Hospital.* London: National Corporation for the Care of Old People.

Nyquist R., Hawthorn P. J. (1987). The prevalence of pressure sores within one health authority. *Journal of Advanced Nursing*, **12**, 183–7.

Pajk M., Craven G. A., Caerson-Barry L. (1986). Investigating the problems of pressure sores. *Journal of Gerontological Nursing*, **12**, 11–15.

Versluysen M. (1985). Pressure sores in elderly patients: the epidemiology related to hip operations. *Journal of Bone and Joint Surgery*, **67B**, 10–13.

Versluysen M. (1986). Pressure sores: causes and prevention. *Nursing*, **3**, 216–18.

Warner U., Hall D. (1986). Pressure sores: A policy for prevention. *Nursing Times*, **82**: 16, 59–61.

8 Drugs and the drug round

The safe administration of drugs has long been part of the traditional nursing role. Doctors prescribe, pharmacists dispense and the nurse gives the drugs to the patient. Gould (1988) considers that the nurse's responsibility includes the safe storage of drugs, maintaining adequate stocks, ensuring that the correct patient receives the correct dose of the correct drug at the correct time and recording all drugs given. The UKCC has enlarged upon this basic set of responsibilities and added extra items, such as requiring the registered nurse to possess a knowledge of side-effects of the drugs she is giving to patients and to be involved in teaching patients about their medicines. Recent UKCC pronouncements to the effect that enrolled nurse training did not qualify enrolled nurses to administer drugs unless they had undergone further training has served to hurt and upset a great many (Jackson, 1988).

It is from this weighty set of responsibilities that the current ritual of the drug round emerged many decades ago and has remained unaltered since the early years of this century. How effective is the drug round at meeting Gould's four key points? Does it ensure that adverse side-effects are monitored and reported to medical staff promptly? Finally, do patients understand their medications so that it is safe for them to take them at home and will do so in such a way as to derive the maximum benefit?

'I'm just going to do the drug round.'
At a time when its leaders claim nursing is moving rapidly towards individualized patient-centred care, the drug round remains as one of the great traditional task-oriented rituals, on a par with the bedpan round and the back round. It's a familiar sight – staff nurse and student trudge round the ward with the drug trolley, taking up to an hour to carry out the round.

Nursing staff may be giving medicines to patients with whom they have had little or no immediate contact. In consequence, they may be unaware that the patient had a sleepless night the night before or has been in pain and needs analgesia. This aspect of the problem has already been reviewed in Chapter 5.

Drugs are often left on the locker in little plastic pots (despite what the procedure manual may say) for the patient to take later, with no way of following up to ensure that they are taken. It is unlikely that the staff nurse will be able to monitor for side-effects if she or he is running a busy 30-bed ward. There simply is not time for her or him to teach all of the patients about the reasons for their medication, how frequently they should take it and what they should look out for by way of side-effects. We would suggest that the drug round makes it very difficult for nursing staff to meet a significant proportion of their responsibilities in drug administration.

However, the senior nurse on duty has certain legal responsibilities as she or he must hold the drug cupboard keys. Not even a doctor, for example, is allowed access to the controlled drug cupboard. The drugs held in there are the registered nurse's legal responsibility. Maintaining adequate stocks is a crucial responsibility, yet large stocks are unnecessary, expensive, and lead to drugs becoming out of date. There should be a policy of minimum safe-stocking rather than stockpiling, and staff should regularly be checking expiry dates. In many areas individual pharmacists check stock levels on wards daily, though this may not be the case in units such as Accident & Emergency. Closer liaison between ward staff and pharmacists has been a welcome development in recent years and is a trend to be encouraged.

There is therefore a central element of nursing responsibility that can only be discharged in the traditional way with a registered nurse responsible for the ward or unit's overall stocks of drugs. However, the traditional two-nurse drug round must be seriously challenged as the best way of giving drugs to patients. Firstly, it is a task-oriented system that does not fit into the ethos of holistic patient-centred care; secondly, it frequently fails to work in practice.

To tackle the first point first, if a single nurse is made responsible for the care of a group of four patients, it is only logical that this care should include the drugs those patients receive. If a student is taken away for an hour to be the checker on the drug round, nobody is caring for her or his patients during that time. It is also of questionable educational value to occupy a student in this way for an hour or so. Even if attempts are made to teach the nurse about the drugs administered on the round, the sheer volume of information with which she or he is bombarded will mean that very little is retained. Further, they are facts in a vacuum, not related to the individual patient and his or her illness, again making learning more difficult.

In an ideal world, each group of patients would have a qualified nurse responsible for them. The drug round could therefore be split into several mini drug rounds with the nurse responsible for those patients administering their medications and then passing the trolley on to the next nurse. It should be noted that there is no legal requirement, except for controlled drugs, that drugs should be double-checked. One nurse acting alone may administer medication (Gould, 1988).

However in the real world, patient allocation usually means that the nurse responsible for several patients is not registered. The compromise therefore should consist of the registered nurse carrying out the round, but the nurse responsible for each group of patients checks the medications with the registered nurse. Thus there are several different checkers per round. The advantage of this system is that drug administration becomes part of the nurse's whole patient care. The registered nurse needs accurate information such as whether the patient feels nauseated, is in pain, or has complained of possible drug-related side-effects. If the second checking nurse has been caring for that patient throughout the shift, the registered nurse is more likely to receive this information. The situation becomes educationally more beneficial to the student as she or he can now learn about drugs a few at a time and can directly relate the drugs to familiar patients and complaints.

Now to examine the second point – how the drug round frequently fails to work in practice.

'I know it's only 6.30, but it's time for your morning pills.'

Stable blood levels of drugs are needed to ensure maximum effectiveness, hence the requirement that they be given in fixed amounts at fixed times. The way many drug administration procedures are timetabled, nurses are required to give patients medication at 0600 hours. This is the source of many problems.

Both authors' experience as Royal College of Nursing stewards leads to the impression that a disproportionate number of reported drug errors occur at this time. Nursing staff will have worked a long night shift and therefore are tired. Research into circadian rhythms indicates that problem-solving ability and mental alertness are at a minimum at 0400 hours and do not improve significantly until well after 0600 hours. There are many tasks competing for the night nurse's attention at this time as she or he tries to get patients up for the arrival of the morning shift. These factors combine to raise the risk of errors to unacceptably high levels if there is a drug round at 0600 hours. This is a ritual that has been abandoned at many hospitals but which remains at many others. It is an invitation to disaster to expect tired night staff to try and carry out a full drug round at this hour; it is a matter of surprise that more errors do not occur.

The true incidence of errors may in fact be significantly higher than is officially recorded, due to nurses simply not reporting errors for fear of the strict disciplinary approach that is usually taken by management. Thus being 'tough on discipline' may be counterproductive, especially as it may lead to nurses who need help and counselling hiding their difficulties with, for example, calculation, for fear of falling foul of the disciplinary process (see below).

A further point concerns the patient's point of view. We will discuss more fully the patient's day in Chapter 11, but many patients have never got up at 0600 hours in their lives, except for special occasions. The drug round ritual ignores the lifestyle of the individual and demands that he or she should be woken at 0600 hours, sometimes even earlier. It is an example of care being tailored to suit the needs of the hospital or nursing staff, not the needs of the patient.

'You failed to give Mr Ryan his frusemide at lunchtime. That's an error which I have to report to the office.'

The timing of the 0600 hours drug round is a prime cause of drug errors. However the ritual of two nurses taking more than an hour to carry out the series of repetitive tasks involved with any drug round is likely to lead to errors at any time of the day. The reason is easy to see as the unstimulating and repetitive nature of the task may lead to the nurse's concentration wandering; the duration of the round is likely to be greater than her or his normal attention span. There are of course other causes of error, such as ambiguous prescribing by doctors, but the ritualistic nature of the round contributes significantly to the risk of errors occurring.

We have advocated breaking the round down into a series of mini-rounds, as this will permit the nurse responsible for a group of patients to be the second checking nurse in the administration of medication. It is likely that the checking nurse in this situation will be more alert and more effective if she or he is only responsible for checking the medication for 4–6 patients who are well known to her or him, rather than checking for the whole ward. Drug errors may be expected to be reduced if such a system was followed.

Once an error has occurred, another nursing ritual takes over – the post-Salmon equivalent of being reported to Matron. Health authorities have drawn up rigid disciplinary procedures and, through the hierarchical system of pre-Griffiths nursing management, they have come to be rigorously enforced.

Crime deserves punishment, nobody would argue with that, but is a human error a crime? Some nurse managers treat it that way, so even the most minor error is the subject of the full majesty of the health authority disciplinary procedure with formal investigatory hearings, written warnings, final written warnings and the rest of the paraphernalia of power and authority. The result is a great deal of stress to already stressed staff who may feel that after all the hard work they have put in, they are entitled to expect better than a harsh, unsympathetic, ritual of punishment for the first minor human error they make.

If management wish to improve staff morale and save a considerable amount of time and money, they should remove drug errors from the category of disciplinary offences. An error certainly must be recorded and the doctor responsible for the patient informed immediately. Once the patient's welfare has been safeguarded attention should turn towards why the error happened rather than a punishment ritual directed at the unfortunate nurse whose only crime has been to be human. Experience indicates that most nurses are terribly upset when they discover they have made an error. If managers wish to cling to the punishment ritual, they should be satisfied with their pound of flesh at that stage. The feelings of guilt and annoyance at oneself that accompany an error are sufficient punishment for most nurses.

A more positive management response would be to find out why it happened. What mistake did the nurse make? In the light of this information, what steps are necessary to avoid repetition? There are a whole range of possible answers from altering unsatisfactory procedures, changing ambiguous drug charts, drawing medical staff's attention to unsatisfactory prescribing, changing drug administration times to improving staffing ratios. The nurse may need counselling, updating of her knowledge or remedial work in maths. All of these are positive responses that acknowledge a drug error as human error, and seek to avoid repetition in the future.

The removal of errors from the field of automatic disciplinary action should open this area up to research. Such research could be expected to make a significant contribution to reducing the frequency of errors, and it would be easier to conduct without the stigma of disciplinary action hanging over all concerned.

Monitoring of errors is essential, as in the rare case where a nurse is unsafe to practice; then evidence will quickly accumulate to this effect. However this should be only a part of an overall policy of monitoring staff performance aimed at picking out staff who are failing to perform at a satisfactory level before any harm is inflicted on patients, not after. The present system often fails to do this as its rigid adherence to disciplinary procedures means that a nurse must first do something wrong. The old cliché about prevention being better than cure is valid when considering nurses and drug errors as much as in any other area of care.

'No, I don't know what pills I'm on. I just take two pink ones in the morning and if I feel like it, a white one at teatime.'
One feature of the present drug round ritual is that it offers little scope to teach patients about their medication. Many patients are on several different medications. Absence of teaching leads to a situation where the patient sits by the bed; several times a day a nurse puts some pills in front of him or her in a little plastic pot, and the patient takes the pills with little idea of what they are called, their purpose, side-effects or desired dose and frequency. Upon discharge the patient will probably be given similar tablets to take home in order to continue the medication which hopefully has improved his or her condition in hospital. However, if the patient is in such a state of blissful ignorance, is it surprising that he or she fails to take the correct pills at the correct time and starts to become confused? Non-compliance is jargon for the patient not taking the medication properly. However, if the medication has not been properly explained to the patient in hospital, it is really not very surprising that the patient makes errors in self-medication after discharge.

The problem is particularly severe in the elderly. Williamson and Chopin (1980) found that 80% of elderly patients admitted to hospital were on medication and Bliss (1981) showed that 10% of admissions to care of the elderly units are associated with iatrogenic drug-related problems. In other words, the medication the patient was taking was contributing to his or her health problems.

A study by MacGuire et al (1987) confirmed that this picture is still a valid one. Studying a sample of 23 patients on an elderly care unit, they found 2 patients admitted because of drug-related problems. Most of this sample were on more than one drug. Some 20% admitted having difficulty with their medication and the rest relied on somebody else to sort things out for them or had evolved idiosyncratic systems of their own of varying degrees of effectiveness.

Patients in this study admitted that they were not taking some medicines because they did not know what they were for. Anecdotal evidence from this group of patients concerning their ability to take medication at home was very worrying indeed. MacGuire et al point out that patients must know the frequencies and dosages of medications because repeat prescriptions (commonly used) fail to have this information on the bottle. Bliss (1981) has shown that half the medicines in the hands of elderly people have only 'as prescribed' written on the label by way of instruction.

The concept of self-medication is a logical solution to this problem. Patients who are being discharged into their own care should be able to demonstrate that they are able to self-medicate before discharge. MacGuire et al (1987) describe a system introduced on their unit whereby selected patients are given medication while they are in the ward and made responsible for taking it themselves. Such an approach is advocated by the Orem self-care model of nursing (Orem, 1985) which, as its name suggests, places great emphasis on the nurse helping the patient to achieve self-care.

Bradshaw (1987) has described a different approach to the problem, involving counselling by both a pharmacist and nurse before discharge. The nurse should also assess the patient's ability to read labels and degree of manual dexterity in addition to the patient's home lifestyle to see if there are any social factors which may interfere with ability to self-medicate successfully. As a back-up to this care, each patient should have a card prepared to take home on discharge. The card should clearly identify all the drugs the patient is taking, including dosage and timing. This is particularly beneficial for relatives and other agencies such as the district nurse. Bradshaw concludes that any doubts that exist about the patient's abilities must be passed on to the general practitioner or other appropriate agency.

The approaches described above are examples of good nursing practice aimed at a rational solution to the problem. Either method will be facilitated with the use of individualized care and the breaking up of the drug round, as suggested earlier, so that the nurse responsible for a patient's care is the nurse giving daily medication. The traditional drug round is a time-consuming ritual that fails to fulfil the nursing responsibilities involved in the administration of drugs.

'Sorry, Night Sister is busy doing the IVs on ward 23 and I haven't got my IV card yet.'

There has been a significant increase in the amount of intravenous (IV) administration of drugs in the last few years. This has led to considerable dispute about the involvement of nurses in this practice, with the result that health authorities have insisted that before a nurse may give drugs intravenously she or he must attend a course in the subject of IV medication.

There can be little dispute about the need for such training in view of the hazards involved with IV therapy. However, once a nurse moves to another health authority, she or he has to retake an IV course and be issued with yet another certificate of competence. This is really a rather ridiculous ritual!

The issuing of such certificates is carried out for other skills not taught as part of basic training, such as suturing and defibrillation. It is an illogical situation that a nurse, having proved her or his competence in one health authority, should be required to repeat the exercise every time she or he moves — as regards some skills, but not others. Why not check that she or he is competent to carry out a bed bath or take a blood pressure when transferring between health authorities? It is just as logical!

The solution lies in an agreement that all health authorities will recognize each other's certificates of competence for skills such as IV therapy. Alternatively, such skills should be included in basic nurse training.

Recommendations for good practice

1. The drug round should be broken up into a series of mini-rounds to allow the nurse responsible for a group of patients to be responsible for their medication. A compromise is suggested on p. 85 in cases where this nurse is not registered.

2. The 0600 hours drug round should be abolished and replaced with an 0800 hours timing.

3. If the agreed procedure for giving drugs has been adhered to, drug errors should no longer be considered disciplinary offences, rather a matter for counselling and prevention. While there is little excuse for failing to check a patient's identity, misreading a badly written script or a calculation mistake are not disciplinary matters, but rather should be the subject of counselling.

4. Patients should be fully educated about their medication before discharge.

5. There should be a nationally recognized criterion for competence to administer IV therapy.

References

Bliss M. R. (1981). Prescribing for the elderly. *British Medical Journal,* **283**, 203–4.

Bradshaw S. (1987). Treating yourself. *Nursing Times,* **83**: 6, 40–1.
Gould D. (1988). Called to account. *Nursing Times,* **84**: 12, 28–31.
Hilgard E., Atkinson R. L., Atkinson R. C. (1987). *Introduction to Psychology.*
New York: Harcourt Jovanovitch Co.
Jackson C. (1988). Tested to the limit. *Nursing Times,* **84**: 15, 18.
MacGuire J., Preston J., Pinches D. (1987). Two pink and one blue. *Nursing Times,* **83**: 2, 32–3.
Orem D. (1985). *Concepts of Practice.* New York: McGraw Hill.
UKCC (1986). Administration of Medicines. A UKCC Advisory Paper. London: UKCC.
Williamson J., Chopin J. M. (1980). Adverse reactions to prescribed drugs in the elderly. *Age and Ageing,* **9**, 73–80.

9 Care of the elderly

The editorial column of the *Nursing Times* was moved to observe in 1987 that the care of elderly people 'remains at best unimaginative and at worst unimaginable'. There are refreshing exceptions to this statement, but .it contains much truth. Many of the problems do stem from shortages of money and resources, but they also stem from shortages of initiative and creative thinking, leading to practice that has institutionalized ritual and perpetrated myth.

With such a vast field to examine, there is only room to look at some of the more glaring examples of the myths that abound amongst nurses and the rituals that are practised upon their elderly patients. Readers should be able to think of many more.

'You can't teach an old dog new tricks.'
Garrett (1985) has picked this out as one of the classic myths surrounding elderly people. It is felt that as people age they are unable to learn new skills or adapt to changing situations and of course that their mental ability declines. It is true that mental abilities requiring speed and extensive use of short-term memory do decline in later life (Hilgard et al, 1987). However, other areas of mental ability show little change with age and the accumulated experience of life may more than compensate for any loss of speed in problem-solving.

There are two significant implications of this myth, the first of which concerns how old people see themselves. As Garrett points out, this myth can become a self-fulfilling prophecy, with the result that elderly people come to believe that they cannot learn new skills. This myth undermines the already threatened self-concept and esteem of an elderly person.

If the nursing staff believe that elderly patients cannot adapt and learn new skills, what effort will they make to involve the elderly in occupational therapy or to provide a stimulating, interesting environment for them? Day rooms on long-stay wards with rows of chairs around the walls, occupied by dozing patients while an unwatched TV drones away in the corner, bear sad testimony to the answer.

If the nurse has such a negative view of the patient, helping to contribute to an equally negative self-concept on the part of the patient, how can therapeutic learning occur? How can a patient with late-onset diabetes be taught to manage the disease or care for an ischaemic limb if patient and nurse both think the patient is incapabe of learning new skills?

'It's disgusting. A man of his age still interested in sex, he's just a dirty old man.'
This is another of the great myths of ageing. It is somehow thought that as people age they lose interest in sex and their sexuality. The need for physical comfort and personal contact does not reduce with age, yet as a person ages it becomes less and less acceptable for these needs to be publicly displayed or met. Sexual activity continues in many people well into the seventh or even eighth decade of life.

Sexuality is a problem with which many nurses have not come to terms in younger patients, so it is not surprising that they fail to appreciate the elderly patient's needs in this area. Elderly patients may feel their sexuality is now inappropriate and withdraw from this area of life as a result of the nursing staff's expectations. Such deprivation is inexcusable.

There are wards for the elderly where patients have a characteristic appearance. There is the dishevelled look of elderly men wearing baggy, open-flied trousers covered in stains and nylon shirts several sizes too big. Then there is the standardized ladies' uniform of open-backed nightdress or loose-fitting Crimplene and Velcro dress which the woman would probably never have bought for herself. Individual men and women have been reduced to institutionalized asexual patients. There are many complex reasons why wards should sink to this level, but a lack of awareness of the patient's sexuality figures prominently amongst such reasons.

'Of course the ward smells of urine. It's a geriatric ward, what do you expect?'
The myth of incontinence runs throughout the care of the elderly. McCarthy (1987) paints a gloomy picture of the chances of changing the attitudes of both staff and patients to the myth that incontinence is unavoidable with age. He considers there is little sign of the commitment necessary to promote continence today or hope for the future – a sad indictment of British health care.

McCarthy describes how younger patients presenting with incontinence are likely to receive better, more positive treatment from the health system, while the elderly fare much worse. This is compounded by the belief amongst the elderly that bladder problems and incontinence are inevitable. They are not.

Data from Thomas et al (1980) indicate that the incidence of incontinence amongst those aged 75–84 is 8% for men and 16% for women, while for the age range 85 and over it is 15 and 16%, respectively. Another way of looking at these figures is to say that approximately 8 out of 9 men and 5 out of 6 women over 75 are continent. With the increasing range of interventions available to support continence or at least minimize the effects of incontinence, there is every opportunity for nurses to help elderly people greatly improve the quality of their life.

Social isolation is correctly seen as a major problem facing the elderly. One major reason for withdrawal from society could well be the shame and embarrassment of incontinence. Attitudes are such that elderly people may not seek help; they are too ashamed to admit this apparent regression to infancy, this loss of control over their bodies. The result is withdrawal and isolation.

To appreciate the fallacy of inevitability, consider the study made by Rantz and Miller (1987) of nursing diagnoses made on 328 long-term elderly patients. Urinary incontinence was listed in 26% of the patients or, expressed another way, three-quarters of a large sample of long-term elderly patients did not have incontinence as a problem. The most common nursing diagnoses are listed in Table 1.

Table 1   Nursing diagnoses in 328 long-term elderly patients

Rank	Nursing diagnosis	Percentage of patients
1	Impaired physical mobility	85
2	Total self-care deficit	66
3	Impaired thought process	60
4	Impairment of skin integrity	48
5	Decreased cardiac output	47
6	Potential for impairment of skin integrity	39

From Rantz and Miller (1987).

One final piece of evidence to challenge this myth comes from Waters (1987) in her detailed follow-up of a sample of 32 discharged elderly patients with a mean age of 82.5 years. Interviewed in their homes 5– 10 days after discharge, 26 of the patients reported they were fully independent in maintaining continence. We will return to Waters' study later.

All the evidence shows that incontinence is certainly a major problem for a significant portion of the elderly population, but not for the large majority. The only inevitability about incontinence is that an attitude of inevitability amongst nurses will adversely affect the care of the elderly.

'It's your age, dear.'

This simple statement embodies two myths commonly found in caring for the elderly. Day (1986) has discussed how hospital nurses fall into the trap of assuming that all elderly people experience a major decline in health due to the ageing process and which is therefore irreversible, while Knowles (1987) has discussed the demeaning language nurses use when talking to the elderly.

Day considers such attitudes as ageism. The analogy is with other '-isms' such as, for example, racism – being derogatory about someone simply because of his or her race. She considers that nurses act in the same way towards the elderly, consigning all minor complaints and symptoms to the simplistic category of being due to the patient's age. This relieves the nurse of the responsibility of having to think about causes or the need to try and help the patient. Nothing can be done, it is all an inevitable part of getting old.

Communicating with this hopeless attitude to an elderly person leads to neglect of health. 'What's the point of giving up smoking at my age?' is the sort of attitude nurses may foster. Such an attitude may also reflect the nurse's views on health and the elderly. A much more positive attitude is called for towards ageing, with an acknowledgement of the importance of health education in this age group. Elderly people can play an active part in community life, leading a rich and rewarding life. Even if an elderly person is frail and needs support and assistance, he or she can still have a good life which is well worth living.

The use of demeaning and childish terms when addressing elderly patients projects the myth that the elderly are childish and regress into infancy. Nurses are prone to use words such as 'dear', 'poppet' and 'sweetie' in caring for the elderly. Such language not only insults the patient; it also, according to Knowles (1987), helps propagate the *Angels* image that many nurses desperately wish to be rid of and helps to undermine the achievements of individualized care.

Knowles asks if nurses use this sort of language to place the patient in the role of child playing to the nurse's mother role. Thus the nurse establishes a controlling position with which she feels comfortable when caring for an adult who may be 60 years her senior. There can be no denying that this is the language of infancy and childhood, yet a major aim of care of the elderly is to promote self-care, independence and avoid institutionalization. Clearly such goals are undermined by this language. Knowles suggests that the familiar nursing abbreviation often encountered in care of the elderly, TLC, really stands for treat like a child rather than tender loving care.

'Meals-on-wheels and the district nurse will take care of her after discharge.'

Hospital nurses discharge patients with varying degrees of insight into the support services available to the elderly in the community and their effectiveness. The notion that all elderly patients will have their needs taken care of after discharge by social services and the community nursing services is a myth.

The work of Waters (1987) casts some light on this problem. She investigated how independent elderly people were in ordinary activities of daily living a week after discharge and how effectively their needs were being met. Of her sample of 32 patients, 26 lived alone. The

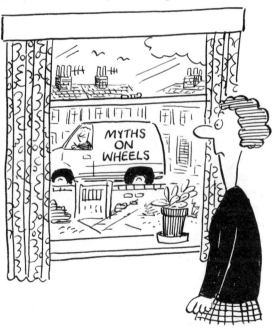

results of her investigation as regards full independence in activities of daily living are given in Table 2.

Did those patients who were unable to achieve independence get the help they needed? A total of 12 out of 32 said they did not. Getting out of the bath was identified as the biggest problem, while half of the sample were seen to be unsteady on walking, even with the use of aids. The patients' ability to manage household chores is summarized in Table 3.

Of the help that was available to patients, 60% was provided by family, 17% by neighbours and friends, 16% by home helps, 6% by district nurses and 1% by meals-on-wheels. Some 80% of help was therefore provided by informal carers – very little by the community nursing service and meals-on-wheels. These figures are in no way a criticism of the community nursing services, rather a realistic reflection of the amount of care they can provide with the limited resources at their disposal. The belief expressed at the start of this subsection – that

Table 2 Number of elderly people who were able to be fully independent in activities of daily living

Activities of daily living	Number ($n = 32$)
Bathing	4
Dressing	25
Continence	26
Toileting	27
Transfer	30
Feeding	30

From Waters (1987).

Table 3 Ability of elderly people to carry out household chores

Chore	Number ($n = 32$)
Heavy laundry	0
Heavy shopping	1
Heavy housework	3
Light shopping	4
Cooking	8
Personal laundry	12
Light housework	13

From Waters (1987).

meals-on-wheels and the district nurse will look after the patient – is therefore seen as the myth it is. It is the large army of unpaid, mostly female, informal carers who provide most of the day-to-day support for the elderly in the community.

The experiences of the group may be summarized by the fact that 20 of the 32 patients felt their independence had been reduced after being in hospital; only 3 reported an increase in independence. Tables 2 and 3 show the reality of how well an elderly person copes after discharge from hospital, and it is rather a different picture from what myth may lead hospital-based nurses to believe.

'She's a bit confused today, though I suppose it's not surprising at her age.'

Confusion and dementia are further examples of the inevitability myths of old age. Because nurses do see many elderly dementing patients, the belief has grown that this too is inevitably a part of ageing. Worse, nurses mix confusion with dementia, with the result that a confused elderly person may be labelled demented.

As Sugden and Saxby (1985) point out, the two conditions are very different. Dementia is sadly a progressive disease with no known medical intervention. However, confusion is usually a short-term problem with a cause that is frequently treatable, such as an acute chest infection, electrolyte imbalance or the psychological effects of sudden hospitaliz-ation.

A confused elderly person is at considerable risk of harm and requires intensive nursing care. However if staff realize the transient nature of the confusion and actively attack the cause of the problem, the patient may be rapidly returned to a normal lucid state. Failure to act swiftly can have disastrous effects: the patient becomes sucked into the hospital system, subjected to increasing doses of tranquilizing medication, labelled as confused with all the stigma attached to such a term, and then falls over and sustains an avoidable fracture of the neck of femur or some other such disaster.

Nurses must clearly differentiate between dementia and confusion, recognizing that the idea that such conditions are inevitable in the elderly is a myth.

In this chapter we have reviewed just a few of the myths associated with age. Recognizing them as myths will go a long way to improving the standards of care received by the elderly in hospital. This should be a major aim of nursing if for no other reason than enlightened self-interest. One day most of us will be old and most of us will die in hospital.

Recommendations for good practice

Nurses should incorporate the following facts into their care of the elderly. An elderly patient:

1. Can learn new skills and be mentally stimulated.
2. Is a sexual being.
3. Will probably be continent.
4. Has reasons for problems that are not linked to age.
5. Is an adult and should be treated like one.
6. After discharge is likely to have significantly reduced independence and will receive only a small proportion of the help needed from official caring agencies.
7. Probably is not and will not become demented.

References

Day E. (1986). Time to value the golden age. *Nursing Times*, **82**: 42, 67–9.

Garrett G. (1985). Ageing and individuals. *Nursing*, **2**, 1230.

Knowles R. (1987). Who's a pretty girl then? *Nursing Times*, **83**: 27, 58–9.

McCarthy C. (1987). Incontinence in the elderly mentally frail. *Nursing*, **3**, 842–4.

Nursing Times Editorial (1987). Editorial comment. *Nursing times*, **83**: 33, 3.

Rantz M., Miller T. (1987). How diagnoses are changing in long term care. *American Journal of Nursing*, **87**, 360–1.

Sugden J., Saxby P. J. (1985). The confused elderly patient. *Nursing*, **2**, 1022–5.

Thomas T. M., Plymar K. R., Blannin J., Meade T. W. (1980). Prevalence of urinary incontinence. *British Medical Journal*, **280**, 1243–5.

Waters K. (1987). Outcomes of discharge from hospital for elderly people. *Journal of Advanced Nursing*, **12**, 347–55.

10 Death and dying

The changing patterns of death in the twentieth century mean that now the vast majority of deaths occur in hospital rather than at home. Most deaths occur amongst people in the age group 55 and over who have usually suffered chronic disease. Sudden death is relatively rare, as is death amongst children. The implications of this for nurses are that they will tend to come in contact with patients who are well advanced in life and whose death is predictable, rather than a sudden event. The major exceptions to this are of course in Accident & Emergency and children's nursing.

Death has been a taboo subject throughout recent history so, not surprisingly, the care of dying patients in hospital has attracted a great deal of myth and ritual to itself. Such practices are not only detrimental to the patient but also to the family and nursing staff. A more open and rational approach to dying has started to develop in recent years, with the hospice movement providing a major impetus to this welcome development. However, the myths remain.

'There is nothing more that can be done for her.'
This comment sums up the negative attitude which many nurses and doctors carry with them when approaching a dying patient. It leads to nothing being done for the patient when in fact there is a great deal that can be done to improve the quality of what life is left to them.

Dicks (1985) argued powerfully against this counsel of despair, pointing out that the provision of adequate symptom control is essential. There is indeed much that can be done to avoid pain, nausea and vomiting, dyspnoea, bowel and urinary disturbance, loss of appetite, coughing, insomnia and confusion, to name just some of the problems faced by the dying patient (Saunders and Baines, 1983).

Dicks argues for the concept of continuing care rather than the traditional staged care model of curative or palliative treatment. This second approach leads to a sudden change in treatment, a change not unnoticed by the patient who may feel abandoned. 'They've given up on me' is a not unnatural feeling. Continuing care is aimed at providing symptom control, rehabilitation, continuity of care and finally terminal care if needed. Curative care is an integral part of this approach but, because of the gradual transition that occurs from a curative focus to symptom control and supportive care, the sudden hiatus between curative and palliative treatment is avoided.

Nurses must believe that symptoms can be relieved before their relief becomes possible. Once the myth of 'nothing can be done' is dispelled and nurses come out from behind the smokescreen of TLC (tender loving care) to assess and tackle individual patient problems positively, then there is much that can be done to improve the quality of the patient's life. Unpleasant and distressing symptoms do not have to be part of the process of dying.

'It will only upset the patient to talk about it.'

Nurses have received little training in the field of communication. Patients with a serious illness tend to ask difficult questions such as: 'It's cancer, isn't it?' or make statements such as: 'I wish it was all over'. The problem is further compounded by the medical convention that only the consultant can authorize telling a patient the truth about his or her illness. The result of this unholy alliance is that nurses desperately try not to talk to patients about death and the nature of their illness. Rationalizations abound, such as the one given above, to justify this behaviour.

This contributes to the 'busy nurse syndrome'; the nurse must keep active, performing tasks at all times, to protect her from the need to talk to patients. When the jobs run out, as they do sometimes despite all the talk of a staffing crisis, what happens? We will answer that question in Chapter 12. For now it is sufficient to say that often little attention is paid to talking to the patients.

Gooch (1988), writing that lack of communication is the cause of most complaints about hospital care, points out how tragic lack of communication can be in the case of care of the dying. Saunders (1978) is even more critical, stating that lack of communication can cause more suffering than many of the symptoms of terminal disease.

It is appalling to say that patients do not want to talk about their illness. It is true that some would rather not talk about it, using denial as a form of defence, but many would, providing they are given the opportunity to do so. Knowing that their questions will get the time and attention they deserve will make it more likely that a patient will talk about his or her illness. Nurses must convey that impression to the patient. If the patient says: 'I would be better off out of it' in the middle of a bed bath, then that is the cue to dry the patient off, stop the procedure and start talking, rather than blandly saying: 'Oh, you'll feel better tomorrow' as you rapidly apply more soap and water to the patient's other leg.

Ufema (1987) presents a series of anecdotal conversations to illustrate how the nurse may skilfully talk to the dying patient, showing this is an essential part of nursing care. Her advice is to be honest and open – this is a nurse's professional responsibility. She is sharply critical of doctors who will not tell the patient the truth and considers that the nurse should seriously question any such deliberate misinformation in just the same way that she or he would question misprescription of a drug. As Ufema points out, she has never been reported by a patient for talking to him or her about dying.

'Have the doctors told the patient yet?'

This often-asked question stems from the fact that some members of the medical profession have taken to themselves the right deliberately to lie in matters of life and death. This monstrous piece of arrogance flies in the face of natural justice, the law of the land and the moral codes of most major religions. What justification then do some doctors have for placing themselves above God and the law? Simply that they know best. What arrogance!

Nurses find themselves trapped by this medical myth when confronted with the difficult question, 'Have I got cancer?', for only the consultant in charge or one of the medical team can answer that question. The unwritten rule is that nurses must only tell patients the same story that the doctor has given; they must defer to the doctor. This leads to the situation that if the doctor deliberately chooses to lie to the patient, the nurse is forced to break her professional code of conduct and collude in deceiving the patient.

What if the nurse should choose to stay with her code of conduct and tell the patient the truth, even though the doctor has said that the patient must not be told the diagnosis? Dimond (1987) has pointed out in a review of the nurse's legal situation that there is an implied term in any employee's contract to the effect that he or she will obey the reasonable orders of the employer. Presumably this includes withholding information from a patient if a consultant has so ordered? Failure to do so is a breach of contract that could lead to dismissal. The question of what is reasonable in this context is highly debatable. A nurse may be faced with the choice of adhering to her code of conduct and being dismissed as a result, or keeping her job by breaking her code of conduct and lying to the patient.

This catch-22 situation seems very unfair on patients and nursing staff. However, given the tradition of nursing subservience to medicine which, as Darbyshire (1987) has argued, is based upon class and gender, it is not surprising. Webb (1987) has rightly argued that knowledge alone does not give a person authority to prescribe how others should behave, neither does gender or class.

Consider the following American example quoted by Webb (1987). A patient asked a nurse for specific information about alternative cancer treatments other than the chemotherapy which the physicians had decided upon. The nurse gave the patient such information and as a result was charged by her state nursing board with interfering in the patient–physician relationship. Judgement went against her and she had to fight her case to the state supreme court to overturn that judgement.

As Webb notes, it would be very interesting to see what attitude the relevant national board would take if a similar case were to occur in the UK. Nurses are legally and professionally accountable for their actions – including deliberately withholding information from patients or even lying to them – so how professionally could a national board pursue a case against a nurse such as the one described above?

As a footnote it is worth looking at a major study by Field and Kilson (1986) which looked at teaching about death in both nursing and medical training. They showed that the subject of death is taught on most basic registered general nurse and enrolled nurse courses. They also found that on average, registered general nurse students spent 50% more time studying the topic than did medical students. Perhaps if doctors are to claim the right to withhold information from a patient about his or her impending death, they should spend at least as little time as other professional groups in exploring the topic at student level.

Consideration of such matters leads to the conclusion that a patient's 'bill of rights' is long overdue; such a bill would guarantee the patient an honest answer to any question asked of a member of staff. It would also make clear once and for all that the nurse must answer questions truthfully and cannot collaborate with the medical profession in deceiving patients.

'It's better for the patient to die at home.'

Dicks (1985) has challenged this widely held belief with the simple question, better for whom? It has been shown that the reason for hospital admission has more often been the relative's difficulties in coping with the advanced stage of the illness, rather than the patient's needs. If continuity of care is to be achieved, the ability of the family to provide care at home must be an essential part of the assessment process. While the individual patient is the focus of care, due attention must be paid to the effects the illness is having on the family. There may be a time therefore when the patient has to be hospitalized for the family's sake.

'Look at me, I'm crying. I'm not hard enough to be a nurse.'

These words were spoken to one of the authors by a third-year student discovered in the sluice, after the death of a child in Accident & Emergency. They convey another myth, that nurses must cover up their feelings or better still, not have any at all.

The nurse with no feelings should not be a nurse, while the nurse who never shows her feelings is probably suffering in other ways that she will not admit. Such suppression of feelings must affect her life adversely; internalizing so much stress must eventually lead to some sort of psychological pathology.

The crucial thing is that feelings and emotions should not interfere with practice, whether in Accident & Emergency or in rational care-planning on the ward. The nurse needs to handle emotions by temporarily putting them to one side in a crisis, but these feelings must be recognized and dealt with afterwards. Situations should be talked through to allow staff – both senior and junior – the chance to verbalize their feelings and emotions.

Certain areas have a relatively high incidence of death, some of which are particularly tragic by nature of the age of the victim or the suddenness of the death. Children's oncology wards, intensive care units and Accident & Emergency are just three examples of areas where support is essential to help staff. Nothing elaborate is needed, just the recognition that by talking about a death, exploring feelings and emotions, nurses can work through their own grieving process. This should be facilitated by arrangements to allow staff perhaps to have a regular working lunch session over sandwiches and coffee, with an agreement that a discussion along these lines will be the starting point for the meeting.

'She'll get over it eventually.'

This is a view often expressed by nurses seeking some crumbs of comfort as they look at a grieving widow on a medical ward or a young woman after an obstetric disaster. The truth is, we do not get over the loss of a loved one, whether it be a husband of 50 years or a fetus of 9 months. The best that can be hoped for is that the person learns to live with the loss and adapts to it. The reader should be sufficiently familiar with the stages of the grieving process to know that the bereaved has a great deal of grief work to perform. It may take many months before he or she can come to terms with the loss, but it remains a loss for all that.

The view that the loss of a fetus is not so serious since the woman never knew the baby as a living human being is a dangerous myth. Lovell et al (1986) demonstrated the depth of grief and mourning felt by mothers in a detailed study of 15 women who had experienced a perinatal death. They all went through the stages of grief, except they had the additional problem of not knowing the life they were grieving over. Strong feelings of guilt were present and an undercurrent of disbelief concerning the various explanations they had been given by the health professionals. Would such women get over these feelings in time?

In another study described by Lovell et al (1986) a sample of elderly women were approached in an investigation of childbirth practices in the early years of this century. Of those approached, 20% declined to take part because they had lost babies and the memories were too painful – half a century later.

One final observation concerns the previously cheerful patient who one day is withdrawn and depressed for no apparent reason. It could be the anniversary of a loved one's death, or the birthday of a deceased spouse. Sensitive enquiry and giving the patient the chance to talk about his or her feelings, if this is indeed the case, constitute good nursing care for this patient.

'Can you see to the last rites for Mr Wilson please, Nurse?'

Death carries many rituals with it in all societies, and the hospital is no exception. The last rites contain many bizarre rituals that have no logical explanation.

The person whose death is expected has usually been transferred into a side ward a few days earlier. This begins the process of isolation. It is easier for the nurse to avoid talking to the dying person if he or she is in a side ward; it is easier not to think about him or her. Is this in some way one of our own defences against death? Watching a person die reminds us of our own mortality; therefore we would rather not see too much of a patient in the last days and hours. This is rationalized by saying that it would be distressing for other patients if they knew someone was dying. Nurses who really believe they can transfer an obviously ill patient into a side ward to die without other patients realizing what has happened are deluding themselves.

After death the body is usually washed. Why? Even if the patient has been bed-bathed only an hour before, this ritual is frequently performed. Chapman (1983) describes nurses wearing gowns to perform this ritual washing, although there are often no cross-infection risks to justify this step. Even if there were, plastic aprons would then be the correct attire. Chapman wondered if the gown was a ritual device to act as protection from distaste and fear of the corpse.

The bed linen is frequently changed, even though it may be perfectly clean, and after removal of the corpse the bed and mattress are scrubbed clean along with the locker and other items in the side ward. There is no rational basis for this ritual. Chapman even describes the mattress being sent for sterilization in some of the hospitals she observed.

The rituals continue, with concealment of the body during removal. Mortuary trolleys are invariably disguised as something else; at one London hospital this ritual is taken to the extent of removing dead babies in wickerwork travelling cat baskets. As the mortuary trolley collects the corpse, it is not uncommon to see curtains pulled around all the beds so the patients cannot see. They can hear, and they can see an empty bed where half an hour ago there was a very sick patient. Most patients realize what has happened, but nobody talks about it. Does this help or hinder the patient who yesterday was told he had cancer or who has just survived his second myocardial infarction? What unspoken thoughts go through his head, giving rise to what anxieties, as the rituals of death are played out before him?

The need is for nurses to adopt a rational policy to the question of death. Nursing must strip away the rituals and look at what lies behind them. What are the fears and anxieties about the death of a patient that lead to such irrational actions? A more rational, caring environment with nurses having insight into their actions might follow from such an exercise.

Recommendations for good practice

1. Nurses should recognize that a great deal can be done for the dying patient to maximize quality of life.
2. Patients should have the right to know the truth at all times about their diagnosis.
3. Nurses should be allowed to be open and honest in talking to patients.

4. Talking about the death of a patient amongst staff should be encouraged as a means of letting nurses do their own grief work. Mutual support groups in high-stress areas should be established.
5. The procedures involved in last offices should be examined in order that ritual can be removed from rational action, and the psychosocial needs of nursing staff can be met in other more beneficial ways.

References

Chapman G. E. (1983). Ritual and rational action in hospitals. *Journal of Advanced Nursing*, **8**, 13–20.

Darbyshire P. (1987). The burden of history. *Nursing Times*, **83**: 4, 32–4.

Dicks B. (1985). Care of the dying cancer patient. *Nursing*, **2**, 1278–9.

Dimond B. (1987). Your disobedient servant. *Nursing Times*, **83**: 4, 28–31.

Field D., Kilson C. (1986). Formal teaching about death and dying in UK nursing schools. *Nursing Education Today*, **6**, 270–6.

Gooch J. (1988). Dying in the ward. *Nursing Times*, **84**: 21, 38–9.

Lovell H., Bokoula C., Misra S. (1986). Mothers' reactions to perinatal death. *Nursing Times*, **82**: 46, 40–2.

Saunders C. (1978). *The Management of Terminal Disease*. London: Edward Arnold.

Saunders C., Baines M. (1983). *Living with the Dying: The Management of Terminal Disease*. Oxford: Oxford University Press.

Ufema J. K. (1987). Dying patients. *Nursing*, Aug, 43–5.

Webb C. (1987). Professionalism revisited. *Nursing Times*, **83**: 35, 39–41.

PART TWO

The Rituals
of Organization

11 The patient's day

Situations can be perceived in very different ways, depending on the observer's point of view. If we apply this statement to a hospital ward and look at the events of a day through the eyes of a patient, we may see things very differently from the normal nursing view. How rational are the things patients are expected to do in the course of a day? What does the ward look like from the patient's point of view? These two questions might best be answered by looking at a 24-hour period on a hypothetical, though typical, ward.

'Wake up, Mr Doyle, it's time for your medicine.'
We have already discussed the ritual of the 6 o'clock drug round (p. 85). The day still starts for most patients at around this time as harassed night staff try and complete for 0600 hours all the 4-hourly observations — some of which are probably unnecessary — give out medications and early morning cups of tea, and tidy up the ward ready for morning staff. If it is a surgical ward with a list that morning, the night staff may also be involved in getting patients ready for theatre.

This is an example of the patient's day being determined by what is convenient for nursing staff rather than what the patient wants. Many people do not get up at 6 o'clock normally, but now they have to. An often heard complaint from patients is that the days seem so long in hospital. No wonder if the mornings start so early.

If the 0600 hours drug round and 4-hourly observations were changed to 0800 hours, with appropriate changes to other timings (1200, 1600 and 2000 hours), the dawn scramble — and with it many errors — could be avoided. Patients whose individual conditions require medication or observations at other times or more frequently would still receive such attention on an individual basis as appropriate.

'Come along to the dining room, Mr Doyle, it's breakfast time.'
Mr Doyle may not normally eat breakfast at 8 o'clock. He may prefer 9 o'clock or he may prefer to sit on his bed in his pyjamas and eat a

bowl of cornflakes. Unfortunately, on some wards the rules of the institution take over and all patients are expected to eat breakfast in the same place at the same time. If we are to pay more than lip service to individualized care, is this justifiable?

Sandford (1987) showed how it was possible to vary meals and meal times in such a way as to restore individuality on a long-stay care ward for the elderly. She was concerned at the poor appetites and the lack of fluid intake of many patients and resolved to attack the problem from the point of view of making meal times more attractive. This meant abolishing many standard ritualistic practices and being innovative. Not all her ideas worked; the elderly men were not impressed with salads ('rabbit food') or wine as a special treat (they wanted beer!), but many did and her work is a splendid example of what can be achieved by recognizing much of the patient's day as the ritualized routine that nurses have allowed it to become. For example, as the kitchens in Sanford's hospital did not require the hot food trolleys back until 1000 hours, this allowed breakfast to become flexible in timing. Where the patient wanted to eat − sitting on the bed or in the dining room − was also left up to the individual's choice.

'We are just going to give you a bed bath, Mr Doyle.'

The ritual of the bed bath is drummed into student nurses in their introductory block. It is true that some patients are unable to see to their basic daily hygiene and therefore need to be washed in bed. Like all aspects of care, this should be individualized to meet the patient's needs, but the way the bed bath is frequently taught, almost by rote learning, ensures it ends up as ritual.

As with dressing techniques, students are taught a series of tasks that must be repeated in a certain order if the students are to be assessed as competent. How much attention is paid to teaching students to assess the needs and wishes of each patient, so that unnecessary ritual is avoided? A good starting point would be to consider whether the patient needs or wants a bed bath. If the answer to either question is 'no', the nurse should not proceed with the full procedure as the patient may be quite happy with washing hands and face.

Experience suggests that some nurses seem almost afraid of using soap to wash patients. It is not uncommon to see the cloth lightly soaped and then rinsed in water, so that the little bit of soap is washed away; then the cloth is squeezed almost dry before the nurse attempts to wash the patient. Does the nurse ask patients how much soap they like to use or at what temperature they would prefer the water? The procedure book often does not acknowledge the patient as having any role in care, apart from being the passive recipient.

Mouth care is another example of ritualistic nursing, as Page et al (1987) showed in their review of the literature on this topic. They demonstrated that most methods of mouth care are traditions with no base in reason or evidence. The faithful glycerin thymol mouthwash tablets have no antibacterial effect; they merely provide a transient refreshing effect. Sodium bicarbonate is ineffective in cleaning the mouth and carries with it the risk of causing chemical burns if the solution is made too strong. How many nurses do know the correct strength? Hydrogen peroxide's bubbling action has been shown to loosen debris, but there is a superior alternative that has been demonstrated to be most effective in tens of millions of people over many decades. This alternative is called toothpaste.

A wide range of implements are used in mouth care. Gauze and cotton wool balls are frequently used but they fray and catch on rough surfaces. They do not dislodge plaque from teeth and need considerable pressure to have any effect on the soft tissues of the mouth. Foam cubes on sticks used in conjunction with solutions can remove debris from soft tissue but not from teeth, while the use of forceps to manipulate any material in mouth care has been condemned by many researchers as totally impractical. The finger with a swab wrapped around it merely compresses plaque between the teeth, is extremely unpleasant for the patient and must carry an unacceptable risk of infection for the nurse. The human bite leads to a very high incidence of infected wounds, whilst the risks of hepatitis and AIDS are also present.

The best implement to use in mouth care is the most obvious – a small soft-bristled toothbrush. Even unconscious patients, provided their airway is protected, can have mouth care with the nurse using a toothbrush, as has been well demonstrated on intensive care units in the authors' experience.

After the bed bath, Mr Doyle will probably have the entire bed changed, regardless of whether it is clean or dirty. Do nurses change the sheets every 24 hours at home? Even ambulant patients have their beds completely remade after stripping down to the mattress. Do nurses do this at home every evening with their own beds? Nurses complain the wards are short-staffed and they do not have enough time to look after patients properly, yet on some wards they find the time to remake completely 30 beds before 10 o'clock every day! There is no justification for stripping and remaking beds in this way, unless the bed linen is dirty.

'Time for your morning bath, Mr Doyle.'

On many wards there is an obsession with putting all ambulant patients in the bath in the morning. How many people normally have a bath in the morning? Insisting on this ritual is another example of not allowing patients to be their normal individual selves. As we shall see in the next chapter, is this the most sensible time to be bathing patients? If there is an afternoon overlap when there are more staff, this time can be utilized for activities such as patient-bathing. Other patients may prefer a bath last thing at night as it relaxes them and helps them sleep.

Bathing patients carries a potential for cross-infection via the bath, especially if broken areas of skin or a catheter are present. Baths are also uncomfortable for some patients to use. More use should be made of showers because some patients prefer them and they are far more hygienic.

'Mr Harris has gone home. Strip his bed down and get it ready for the next admission.'

Stripping and replacing the linen is rational, but is washing the mattress? Yet another meaningless ritual involves washing the mattress with a variety of solutions from soap and water to spirit. Apart from wasting nursing time (do you wash the mattress at home every time you change the bed?), this procedure damages the mattress. The outer cover loses any waterproof properties it may have and the mattress gradually becomes a wet sponge, soaking up urine, vomit, wound discharge, spilt tea and soup and of course more water next time it is washed after another patient has gone home. The plastic keeps it dry on the outside, but inside there is a positive bacterial broth stewing away with great scope for cross-infection. An infection control officer recently told one of the authors that she was no longer worried about the absence of flame-retardant covers on mattresses because there was so much water in them that if there was a fire, throwing ward mattresses on it would be the best way of putting it out!

'I wonder why Mr Doyle looks so worried?'

There are many reasons why a patient may be sitting at his bedside in the afternoon looking worried. Maguire (1985) has shown that psychological and social problems remain unidentified by nurses in up to 80% of physically ill patients. Nurses wrongly assume that patients will reveal these problems without prompting.

Accounts by patients of their hospital experiences offer insights into their fears and anxieties and should be carefully studied by nurses. Lack of communication is a constant theme – either nobody tells the patient why things are happening or only a half-complete explanation is given. Two such accounts are by Holgate (1988) and Mallows (1985). Holgate describes feeling isolated and vulnerable after his coronary artery bypass surgery. He was surprised to find how reassuring it was to be touched by nurses, even when they were carrying out tasks such as observations. Touch is very culture-dependent and in British culture it is rather frowned upon. One day Holgate found himself sat up in bed, crying for no reason. Several nurses sped past the end of his bed looking very embarrassed before one asked him what was the matter. When he said it was nothing, he couldn't understand why he was crying, she merely said it was 'quite normal' and walked away. There was no explanation; the patient was merely told that something he considered to be abnormal was quite normal!

Mallows (1985) gives a dismal account of the lack of communication surrounding his stay on a trauma ward after he had sustained a head injury which required neurosurgery to relieve an intracranial haematoma. The communication failures ranged from not even being told which hospital he had woken up in (he assumed it was his local hospital, which led to him giving incorrect answers when asked if he knew where he was) through to an explanation from a junior doctor as to the mechanism of his brain injury which he realised defied the laws of physics (he was a lecturer in mechanical engineering)!

Accounts such as these report that nursing staff seemed to be very busy with their physical care – for which the patients are grateful – but without communicating. It is almost as if being in hospital is a game in which patients have to work out for themselves what is happening and why, as nobody will tell them.

Good communication, giving patients information and explanations, will benefit their progress in many ways. Anxiety and worry are likely to breed in the fertile soil of ignorance. If nurses wish to have patients cooperate fully with care, then nursing's side of the bargain must be to tell patients exactly what is happening and why in a language they can understand. Compliance requires communication. If care is to become patient-centred it must involve the patient in the planning stages. This will only occur if nurses communicate with patients instead of going about ritualistic tasks or procedures learnt by rote.

'Lights out now, it's 10 o'clock.'
At the end of the day Mr Doyle will be confronted by what both Mallows (1985) and Holgate (1988) thought of as the worst part of

hospitalization – the night. The rituals continue with lights out well before most patients normally go to bed at home.

Mallows recalls feeling very alone, hearing strange sounds yet seeing little of the nursing staff, while for Holgate the nights were very long. He felt that the nursing staff were totally untrained in handling distress or caring. The noises of the ward and the heat and light made sleep very difficult. Minor things were magnified as he lay there with nothing to occupy his mind and unable to sleep.

Hilton (1987) has shown just how noisy hospitals can be, finding that hospital noise levels frequently exceed the maximum permitted, adding considerably to the patient's stress. Holgate (1988) monitored sound levels in four intensive care and two general wards, using microphones and tape recorders. The worst offenders were the postop recovery room and the intensive care unit of the largest hospital in the study. Loud talking by staff, movement of chairs or stools, bedrails being put up and down, alarms, ripping paper and even the use of dustbins generated more noise than everybody's favourite culprit, the phone. Many patients who had been through these two wards were very critical of the noise levels when interviewed later.

How sensitive are night staff to the individual needs of patients? Many try to talk to patients about their feelings at night, but with staffing levels as they often are, this is difficult. Individualized care in terms of talking to patients is made more difficult as it may disturb other patients who are trying to sleep. However, if the ward has a day room this offers a solution to the problem. Nurses should try, despite the difficulties, to practise individualized care on a 24-hour basis.

Recommendations for good practice

1. Evaluate various routine tasks. Are they necessary?
2. Ask patients what they think about their stay in hospital. This should be part of an on-going quality control programme. A health authority could employ a quality control officer to interview a sample of patients at home between 1 and 2 weeks after discharge. Feedback on the patient's perceptions of hospital life should allow nurses to make their care better and more patient-centred.

References

Hilton A. (1987). The hospital racket. *American Journal of Nursing*, Jan, 59–61.
Holgate R. (1988). In the small hours. *Nursing Times*, **84**: 21, 34.

Maguire P. (1985). Consequences of poor communication. *Nursing*, **2**, 1115–18.
Mallows D. (1985). Communication, a patient's view. *Nursing*, **2**, 1112–14.
Page C., Sammon P., Shepherd G. (1987). The mouth trap. *Nursing Times*, **83**: 19, 25–7.
Sanford J. (1987). Making meals a pleasure. *Nursing Times*, **83**: 7, 31–2.

12 The nurse's day

Nursing is still largely a female profession, so this chapter will start by looking at how being female influences a typical nursing day. The female nurse's shift begins when she puts on her uniform: the dress, which many nurses admit is impractical for lifting, the belt, badge and stripes that give it all such a military flavour and the cap and apron, the Victorian emblems of servility that serve no practical purpose. These are the components of a typical uniform, all conveying the origins of nursing. Its wearing can only be called a ritual, as rational considerations of the uniform's function should lead to radical changes. Such a review has led areas such as mental illness and mental handicap largely to abandon uniforms.

In debating the issue of uniform, Sparrow (1987) has suggested that the three reasons usually advanced in favour of traditional uniform – identity, cleanliness and freedom of movement – are fallacies.

Patients are confused by the multiplicity of uniforms, rather than assisted, in identifying who is the sister and who is the student. Poor laundry services are cited as leading to nurses failing to change their dresses each day while the freedom of movement afford by an A-line dress and belt is seriously doubted by Sparrow.

If nurses are trying to create a normalizing, caring atmosphere for patients in areas such as care of the elderly, then the wearing of a uniform only undermines such aims by reminding patients of their institutionalized status. A uniform helps to place a barrier between nurse and patient. In more acute general areas, the wearing of traditional uniform fosters the traditional 'angels/naughty nurses' stereotype that most female nurses find so nauseous. It also interferes with lifting, thus endangering the nurse's back. Finally, in the case of the national uniform, it poses a significant fire hazard. More practical uniforms incorporating trousers and a short jacket and dispensing with the belt and cap would seem a welcome development, both in terms of improving patient care and getting rid of the stereotyped public images of nurses. Such a development would also allow male and female nurses to wear the same clothing – a subtle but important step in getting rid of the sexist notion that a man who happens to be a nurse is in some way a different sort of nurse to a woman. Men resent being called 'male nurses'; they are nurses in exactly the same way as their female colleagues.

'Time for report.'

The nurse's day on the ward starts with the ritual of a report. In a traditional ward report she or he will be given a mass of information about all the patients on the ward, regardless of whether she or he is looking after them or not, rather than specific information on the patients allocated to her or him (assuming some sort of patient allocation is practised; see Chapter 16). This report can occupy a whole shift of nurses for up to an hour, especially at lunch time, so that early shift nurses may not go to lunch until after 1330 hours.

We have an inefficient system which is a hangover from the past; in other words, a ritual. If the ward is task-centred, the nurse in charge is the only person who may know what is happening and therefore the full report is needed. How effective is such a report? Lelean (1973) in a classic piece of research showed that the meaning of the sister's instructions could not be interpreted with reliability; verbal reports did not augment written Kardex instructions and could contradict them, while an instruction could have three different meanings on the same ward on the same day. One such verbal instruction, 'up and about' was shown to have eight different meanings to different nurses.

If patient allocation or team nursing is used, the system is still inefficient as nurses sit listening to information about patients they will not be caring for. Worse, the nurse conveying that information may not have cared for any of those patients on the shift just ending if team leaders are not involved in the report-giving.

Another ritual involves the little nursing notebooks in which students usually desperately scribble notes in the hope of being able to retain some shreds of information relevant to their patients. Experience shows that what is written is usually illegible, contains some bizarre spellings as students grapple phonetically with technical terms and abbreviations, and casts little light upon the patient's needs for that shift. Some wards ban these notebooks. They should not be necessary, as theoretically, all a nurse needs to know is written in the care plan. This is a theme to which we will return in Chapter 16.

A much more efficient use of time would be to have a bedside report during which the nurse responsible for a group of patients hands over to the nurse on the next shift. In this way, three or four reports are given simultaneously, cutting time down to perhaps 10–15 minutes and saving several nursing hours. The nurse in charge of all the patients on the shift has an overall handover to the next nurse in charge, concentrating on the important aspects of patient care. In view of the seniority of the nurses and their knowledge of the patients this should not take long.

Experience of working with student nurses shows that they retain very little of significance from the traditional report. This is an area waiting to be researched, together with the number of nursing hours consumed in this way. There must be a more efficient method of passing on patient information than the present ritual.

'Go for coffee when all the baths are done.'

A fascinating ritual of ward life is the way nurses seem preoccupied with 'getting all the work done by lunchtime'. This leads to staff rushing around carrying out dressings at a time when the airborne bacteria count is at a maximum after all the beds have been (ritualistically) stripped and remade. Observations and drugs rounds are crammed in, while the patients must all be up, washed and bathed before high noon brings the lunch trolley wheeling on to the ward.

The results of this ritual are patients who have not received correct care because there was not time and tired staff who are too busy to talk to patients and who do not get to lunch until after 1330 hours. This morning's frantic activity is followed by an afternoon when staff have little to do. If a constructive afternoon programme of teaching aimed at patients and students was organized and staff saw this as a time to talk to their patients, there might be some justification for the morning's frenetic pace, but this is often not the case.

The ward day could be organized much more rationally with the work tailored to maximum staffing times in the afternoon. If nurses practised individualized care, for example, fewer patients would need bathing (or a shower) in the morning as they might prefer the afternoon or evening, and that preference could be satisfied. Fortunately, a lot of wards now carry out dressings in the afternoon rather than the morning. Factors such as whether the wound needs dressing and the best availability of nursing staff taken into account together with minimum air contamination should determine dressing times. Afternoons are more logical in this respect.

The presence of a ward routine timetable pinned up on the sluice wall detailing what should happen when, for all patients presumably for every day of the year is a sad reminder of how rituals are propagated and individualized care is subordinated to institutionalization. Such daily routines may still be found in large, acute general hospitals.

The value of abolishing fixed routines and doing things in the patient's time, of communicating with the patient and taking the patient on board in the care-planning process is well shown in a report by Swaffield (1988) of an experimental ward where such steps have been taken. This study demonstrated that such things are possible, and on a lower staff–patient ratio than many of the wards in the particular hospital studied.

'At least with work books you know the work gets done.'

The work book is a tradition of the task-centred ward that still persists today. Each day, lists of patient names are drawn up under various tasks such as '4-hourly obs' or '2-hourly turns'. The nursing staff work from these lists to ensure that all the tasks are properly done. The research carried out by Lelean (1973) showed that the notion that such patients actually received the care was often a myth on the six typical wards that she studied.

Only 5% of patients who had written instructions for 2- or 4-hourly turning actually received this care. The time between 4-hourly observations was rarely anywhere near 4 hours and could be as little as 80 minutes. If patients required assistance to get in and out of bed, the time they were left out of bed depended on ward routine, not their needs. One final finding concerned the length of time patients were left out of bed; it frequently exceeded the written maximum by 2 hours or more.

This shows the effects of a task-centred approach based on the traditional Kardex. In Chapter 16 the controversy surrounding the nursing process approach to care will be explored, but findings such as these demonstrate that the notion that all is well with the traditional approach is a myth.

'Look, we're really short-staffed this morning, although there were plenty on duty yesterday. I can't understand why.'

The nursing off-duty rota consumes much senior nursing time, and for all that, many wards still seem to suffer a feast-or-famine syndrome. The problem may be made worse by cost-conscious management seeking to reduce the number of relatively highly paid staff who are on duty in the evening and weekends and thus attracting unsocial-hours payments.

Lelean (1973) noted that the number of nurse hours available to patients was unrelated to the ward workload, and that the workload between wards in the same hospital varied enormously. As we move into the 1990s, her comments still ring true as many wards fail to use a rational approach to off-duty and managements fail to carry out realistic patient dependency audits. The shortage of recruits that is now hitting nursing, combined with the disgraceful underfunding of the National Health Service by Government, combine to exacerbate the problem.

Sisters can no longer rely on an ad hoc system of doing the off-duty, often based on ritualistic assumptions. Staffing numbers must be matched to workload. The first requirement is therefore to see how workload varies day by day, shift by shift. Surgical wards need to look at operating days for consultants with beds on their ward, Accident & Emergency units need to look at patterns of attendance. Only when such day-to-day patterns have been established can the next step be taken of evaluating how the workload can be distributed rationally within the day. It is on the basis of such data that an off-duty rota can be drawn up which repeats itself over a set period of weeks, thus allowing staff to know their off-duty several weeks in advance. The hand-to-mouth ritual of doing the off-duty this week for next is unfair to staff and unlikely to produce optimal staffing levels for patients' needs.

'It's night staff's fault.'

This comment sums up the gap between night and day staff. Scott (1988), describing the results of a major study undertaken in 1986 into

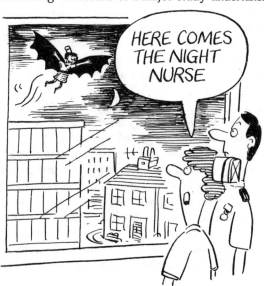

night duty, points to this gap as a major problem. Only one hospital in this study carried out internal rotation, leading to the inevitable 'them and us' syndrome. If patient care is a 24-hour responsibility, can this division be justified?

The lack of in-service training among night staff was highlighted by this study, suggesting that night staff may not be as up to date as they should be with new developments. Night staff felt they were excluded from developments and initiatives were imposed upon them. However, given the management style of some health authorities, day staff probably feel the same in many areas.

The rituals of night duty are ingrained in some nurses who have not seen a ward by day for many years, while for day staff, night duty may only be a dim and distant memory of far-off training days. Is this likely to lead to the best integrated 24-hour nursing service possible? There are strong arguments for internal rotation. It should be acknowledged that there are many part-time staff for whom internal rotation would not be possible since they have small children. Alternatively, more flexible shift patterns should be investigated for such women, such as a twilight shift from say 1800 to 2300 hours. One drawback is that women would need their own transport due to the lack of public transport at such times and the risk to personal security involved in a woman walking home at that late hour.

The introduction of the Project 2000 reforms has major implications for the night staffing of many areas, as at present many wards depend heavily on students for their night staff. Night duty clearly shows students as the cheap labour they all too often are. Their large-scale removal from the wards is inevitable, with perhaps each student spending no more than a week or two on nights as part of their 18-month common foundation programme. This is an aspect of Project 2000 that needs urgent attention if serious problems are to be avoided with staffing the wards at night.

The division of nursing into day and night staff is a tradition that must be broken down in the interest of patient care, and to benefit those who are currently disadvantaged on nights. Attendance at study days, conferences or professional development courses is even more difficult for night staff than it is for day staff. There is no single simple way of achieving this integration. Blanket edicts abolishing night duty and forcing all staff on to internal rotation would be met with fierce and justifiable opposition by staff unions. Flexibility, sensitivity and creativity are essential characteristics of any solution to such a complex problem.

It may be concluded that while many individual tasks within the nurse's day are rituals, so too the overall framework of that day, down to the very clothes worn by the nurse, are all part of a bigger ritual – the ritual of nursing.

Recommendations for good practice

1. Research is required into an alternative, more practical nursing uniform.
2. Ward reports should be divided into concurrent team reports.
3. Workload should be linked to the number of staff on duty at any given time rather than ritual and routine.
4. Off-duty rotas should reflect workload patterns and should be planned well in advance.
5. A greater integration of day and night nursing care should be a major goal, using internal rotation only where appropriate, and other flexible shift patterns. Joint staff meetings would further help day and night integration.

References

Lelean S. (1973). *Ready for Report, Nurse?* London: Royal College of Nursing.
Scott E. (1988). Lighting up the darkness. *Nursing Times,* **84**: 21, 28–30.
Sparrow S. (1987). The case against. *Nursing Times,* **83**: 15, 41.
Swaffield L. (1988). Tuned in. *Nursing Times,* **84**: 23, 28–31.

13 Hierarchy and autocracy

There is no doubt that nursing is a very hierarchical profession, from the most junior student nurse with her single stripe up to senior ward sisters and beyond. Where does this structure come from and what part does it play in propagating myths and rituals?

As an organization grows, certain functions and the people responsible for them come to be seen as more important than others. Thus a hierarchy evolves with lines of responsibility and control running up and down, which leads to the development of line management, as it is known.

If we are to begin to understand the way that nursing hierarchies have evolved then we must look to the origins of nursing and place them in a historical and social context. These origins lie in both military and religious spheres; consequently, the hierarchical system should come as no surprise, with the development of ranks with titles such as sister and matron. Such titles are of course very sexist – if words in current usage such as *spokesman* are changed to *spokesperson*, then so too the title *Sister* is in need of revision to rid it of its sexist connotation. There is more to it than that, however, for the time of Nightingale was the time of Victoria and Victorian values, which placed great emphasis on the man as the natural head of the family. The woman was subservient to the man and was supposed to be under unquestioning obedience to orders.

The male doctor therefore saw it as natural to tell the subservient female nurse what to do, and she complied, complete with the great Victorian badges of servitude, the cap and apron, so beloved of nurses even today, as shown by their obsession with uniforms. Orders were to be obeyed, not questioned, so the good nurse did what she was told. Subservience to doctors, to men and to anybody in authority, along with a rigid hierarchy, are all part of the legacy of Nightingale and the Victorians which has been handed down to nursing today.

The nursing hierarchy has undergone two major changes in the twentieth century, firstly with the Salmon report which rationalized senior nursing management and created a series of tiers of senior nursing posts above sister level, and then with the recent Griffiths report and the advent of general management, which has removed all the nursing management structures set up by Salmon.

Many in nursing saw this as a direct attack upon the power base built up by nurse managers in the post-Salmon era, a base founded upon the large numbers of nurses and the huge budgets that went with such a labour-intensive profession. Whatever the arguments, it is now history and, despite the fierce opposition of the Royal College of Nursing, nursing has to live with general management.

Within the traditional hierarchy, the manager of a nurse was always a nurse, so professional responsibility stayed within the profession. This no longer happens and sisters may now find their immediate superior in the hierarchy is not a nurse and has little insight into nursing care. This can result in a great deal of friction and disharmony.

Griffiths means that there is now a hierarchy of managers, except they are no longer responsible for managing discrete groups of staff. Glennerster et al (1986) thus see general management as challenging the logic of professional independence within the National Health Service. They recognize that there is a major dilemma which has not been resolved: how can control of nursing by a general manager ensure that effective nursing standards are met if that person is not a nurse?

Inherent in this question is the assumption that in the past nurse managers did maintain high standards of care. While many did, there is also a strong suspicion that many did not. They rapidly became separated from, and out of touch with, clinical nursing, leading to a loss of clinical credibility in the eyes of practical nurses. The rigid hierarchy of nursing however concentrated power in the hands of its managers, leading to frustration amongst clinical staff who were unable to change things. Poor nursing managers came to mean poor nursing care.

There was therefore an element of fantasy in the arguments of some nurse managers that general management would reduce standards, as the nurse managers were so out of touch with clinical nursing that they would not know what represented a good standard of care!

There is an answer to this problem, and that is the widespread establishment of clinical nurse specialists. Such nurses should not be nursing officers by another name, rather they should be clinical nurses with expert knowledge who are able to practise, advise on or teach clinical nursing to the highest standards. Depending on their clinical area they could be responsible for a ward or unit or they might act across the whole hospital, as a stoma specialist does. Not only can such a nurse set standards, but by the vigorous pursuit of quality control and evaluation of care, she or he can be responsible for ensuring that standards, once set, are maintained.

The major regrading exercise of 1988, despite the disruption it has caused in some areas due to unfair and illogical application, offers a wonderful opportunity to clinical nursing as it now makes it possible for such posts to be created and the staff holding these posts to be paid according to their expertise. It is to be hoped that future generations of nurses do not look back and see that such a splendid opportunity was squandered amongst a welter of bickering, jealousy and intransigence.

There is of course a hierarchy within the ward itself from sister down to first-year student. This is based on authority and power, but what underpins that power?

An interesting analysis is provided by Schein (1970) who talks of three types of organization. Firstly, authority may be enforced through pure coercive power (e.g. prisons); then there are organizations which elicit involvement of subordinates by the use of financial rewards and which are based on a rational legal authority (e.g. business and industry). The third category depends upon normative rewards, by which the author means that the opportunity to perform a function brings with it rewards. It is the value of the function itself that provides the reward, not money, and the hierarchy is sustained within this value system. This third group includes hospitals and religious orders.

The hierarchy of the ward is sustained by this latter system, with high-prestige jobs such as doctor's rounds and technical tasks being carried out by sister or the senior staff nurse and low-prestige jobs such as cleaning the sluice by a first-year student. Turnock (1987) discusses how nurses themselves see some tasks as having more prestige than others. It is regrettable to hear nurses talking of 'basic nursing care' as some low-order task fit for unqualified auxiliaries and junior students, because from the patients' point of view such basic care is the highest priority. One could also ask, what is basic care, if not the very essence of nursing? However, it is the ability to perform an electrocardiogram or some other hi-tech procedure that is rated highest and ensures for its practitioner a place at the top of the ward hierarchy.

The hierarchy puts a leader at its head, whether the ward sister or the general manager. What sort of leadership style will that person adopt? The burden of history often leads to an authoritarian or autocratic style in nursing, although there are welcome exceptions.

Sullivan and Decker (1985) characterize autocratic leaders as those who make decisions alone. They do not consult and so lack group support; they direct and tell others what to do rather than ask their opinions first. They tend to be more concerned with task accomplishment ('getting the work done') than with any concern for those performing those tasks. They expect orders to be obeyed and are characterized by having little trust in junior staff, who are thought of as irresponsible or lazy. Further traits described include being resistant to change and indifferent to organizational needs.

We would wager that the reader will immediately be thinking 'that reminds me of...'. This authoritarian style fits well into the nursing traditions of unquestioning obedience and servility inherited from Nightingale's Victorian ladies.

Having discussed hierarchies and autocracy in general terms, it now remains to look at how they affect nursing today, for we contend they are largely instrumental in propagating much of the ritual and mythology discussed in this book so far. A good place to start is the area where students learn – the school of nursing.

Various writers have argued that traditional schools of nursing compare unfavourably with other adult education institutes. The views of Gooch (1984), for example, to the effect that tutors tended to have a 'schoolmarm' approach to students who they believed would act irresponsibly with less supervision (autocracy in action!) produced a defensive response from a group of tutors (Wrigley et al, 1984) who were unable to discuss the criticisms rationally; they merely defended what they were doing.

It is certainly the experience of nursing in higher education that students can be given the freedom to be responsible for their own learning. There are approximately 20 university and polytechnic-based honours degree courses in nursing in the UK, and students on these courses tend to follow a very different educational path from their colleagues in many traditional National Health Service schools of nursing.

It would be a mistake if nursing were to regard graduates as some sort of élite. Commonly heard myths suggest that graduate nurses are all theory and no practice or that they are only doing a degree so they can become managers. Both statements are wrong.

To take the first point, graduate nurses have satisfied the minimum number of hours of practical experience required by the UK statutory bodies and also the European Community. While registered general nurse students do have more practical hours' experience, a large proportion of those hours (such as night duty) cannot be called educationally beneficial as the student is in fact only a pair of hands. Developing the argument further, it is true that undergraduate students do study a lot of theory, but if a nurse does not understand the theory of care, what has she or he got to base her or his care upon other than the sort of rituals and myths identified in this book? Lack of factual knowledge will lead to poor nursing care and it is the authors' experience that those undergraduate students who are the best academically are at least as good as the best registered general nurse students when it comes to practical nursing care.

With regard to the second point – that all graduate nurses want to be managers – follow-up studies show that a graduate nurse is more likely to be clinically employed than health authority trained RGNs. They do not become managers but stay in the clinical field – a trend that will probably be amplified as a result of the new clinical grading structure.

Nursing would therefore be making a major error if it was side-tracked into status arguments comparing registered general nurses and undergraduate trained nurses. The truth of the matter is that nursing needs both types of student, and if the general thrust of Project 2000 is towards the academic model of higher education, then nursing must realize that this is the right road to go down if we are to produce a professional workforce with the skills necessary to delivery quality nursing care in the future.

Opposition to academic developments in nursing probably stems from the insecurity of non-academic nurses and the threat they perceive from such students. Experience shows that undergraduates have a lot to learn from registered general nurses and that the converse is also true. The freewheeling, questioning, self-directed learning approach that characterizes higher education will present traditionalists with a major challenge, but it is interesting to note that in the authors' experience there are many registered general nurse students who, having worked alongside and become friendly with undergraduates, have expressed a preference for that model of training over their own traditional registered general nurse course.

Johnson (1986) describes schools of nursing as bureaucratic institutions with strong patterns of authority and a clear-cut hierarchy from clinical teachers and tutors up through senior tutors to director of nursing education level. This leads to students' problems frequently being dealt with at an inappropriate level as the responsibility passes up the line of command to senior tutor level at least before any executive action can be taken. This buck-passing delays action and leaves the student facing a senior tutor she or he probably does not know. A stranger who is also a clear representative of authority, blessed with the power to hire and fire, is perhaps not the most appropriate person for a student nurse to discuss her or his problems with.

The use of disciplinary procedures by senior tutorial staff against students is totally inappropriate. Invoking health authority procedures that were drafted with serious offences such as theft in mind, for use in an educational setting is unacceptable. Hierarchies do not like being challenged and the student who does not conform quickly finds her- or himself the subject of disciplinary action. It is all very well for the director of professional conduct for the UKCC, Reg Pyne, to state that nurses should speak up against conditions that threaten patient care (Pyne, 1987), except that when they do so, they frequently find the full weight of the health authority disciplinary procedure against them.

What is their offence? A breach of confidentiality, according to health authorities. The clause inserted in contracts of employment about confidentiality rightly seeks to protect individual patients' privacy; it is not there to be used as a weapon by authoritarian managers who twist the meaning to include anything the person sees or hears of during daily work. Thus the student who speaks out as an individual to the press about dangerous staffing levels will find that she or he is in dire disciplinary trouble. The citing of this clause is beginning to become more widespread and it has recently been used by the Bath health authority against a doctor who spoke out against conditions.

In moving from the sublime to the ridiculous, one further example will suffice, and it is given by Johnson (1986). It is the story of how a student was considered by a senior tutor to be lucky only to be given a final written warning after accepting a psychiatric patient's invitation to share a piece of bacon at breakfast time. The student had been charged with theft of hospital property!

Such petty-minded and authoritarian attitudes amongst nurse educators led Johnson to a powerful plea for a move away from the traditional authoritarian school to a more humanistic approach, characteristic of other areas of adult education. If students learn their nursing in the sort of atmosphere that sees failing an exam as a disciplinary matter, and accepting a piece of bacon from a patient as an act of theft warranting dismissal, it is difficult to see how they will become the thinking, questioning nurses of tomorrow. Project 2000 offers a splendid opportunity for nursing, but are there enough nurse educators with the vision to make it work?

The problem of hierarchies was intimately involved in the 1988 regrading exercise. The principle aim was to create a series of salary bandings that would fairly reward nurses for responsibility and experience. The end product was a bitter dispute and industrial action which included the concept of 'working to grade'. This led to reports of intensive care unit nurses at a prominent children's hospital refusing to carry out physiotherapy on their patients while other nurses refused to take patients to the toilet without registered nursing supervision. Such acts not only harm patients but do fundamental damage to the notion of professionally maintained standards of nursing care. It will be a sad reflection on nursing if the only result of the regrading exercise is the establishment of a rigid new hierarchy based on grade letters, D nurses and F nurses, A nurses and I nurses, with a whole new plethora of badges of rank and privilege.

The notion of hierarchies can also be extended into the rivalry between nurses, midwives and health visitors. Midwives see themselves as different from nurses, being practitioners in their own right. Cynics might say that midwives see themselves as superior to nurses. The tensions and jealousies between such groups came close to wrecking the legislation that led to the formation of the UKCC and the national boards and it has simmered away ever since, resurfacing in the 1988 regrading dispute. Attempts to set up interprofessional hierarchies ignore what is best for the patient and have more to do with personal prestige than patient care.

An interesting insight into how hierarchies function on wards comes from Lelean's work (1973). She found that sisters spoke to first-year students for only 2% of their available time or, expressed another way, on at least half of her days on duty, the sister did not speak to a first-year student and on just over a third of days she did not speak to a nursing auxiliary. Of the conversations that the sister held which were over 1 minute in length, 60% were with registered nurses and 3% with junior students. On average the sister would speak for 40–50 minutes per shift with medical staff.

These figures reveal the effect of rigid hierarchies in isolating the leader, the sister, from junior students. Thus the person who should be a powerful role model for students is diminished; the importance of this will be seen in the next chapter. It confirms the suggestion that hierarchies are built upon the perceived importance of tasks. Talking to doctors is seen as an important, high-value function so this role is carried out by the sister. It should also be noted that there are many consultants who will only speak to the sister, but this will be discussed in the next chapter.

The sister is the senior clinical nurse with the most experience and the nurse who carries the responsibility for the nursing care on a ward.

The junior students and nursing auxiliaries are the nurses who have most patient contact. Consideration of the figures in Lelean's (1973) study therefore reveal a major problem; how can the sister know what is happening and how can she influence care if she has such little interaction with the staff carrying out the bulk of the care? It is also possible to question seriously the learning environment of such a ward, for how are the students to learn from senior nursing staff if they never talk to them?

Problems such as these flow logically from a task-centred, hierarchical model of care. A twin approach is therefore needed. Firstly individualized care and primary nursing should replace task-centred care, and secondly the rigid hierarchies need to go. The sister should be acknowledged as a democratic team leader, rather than an autocrat. Her clinical expertise should command respect rather her grade G demand it. She should see herself as a facilitator of nursing care planned on a primary nursing basis by her trained staff. Her role becomes one of teaching and advising, leading by example by actually carrying out nursing care where necessary, and providing the right atmosphere and resources to optimize patient care. If the reader thinks this is not possible, consider the role of a typical hospital consultant; it is not that dissimilar. Consider also the wisdom of Lao Tsu; 'To lead the people, walk behind them' or, expressed another way, 'True leadership must be for the benefit of the followers not the enrichment of the leaders. In combat, officers eat last' (Townsend, 1970).

Recommendations for good practice

1. Schools of nursing need to practise a more humanistic approach to education, starting with removing students from the health authority disciplinary code. This will have to happen with the implementation of Project 2000 as students will no longer be employees of the authority.
2. Primary nursing should be implemented.
3. Democratic leadership styles should be taught to students as part of the hidden curriculum of their training, while first-line management courses should be structured around fostering this concept.

References

Glennerster H. et al (1986). *The Nursing Management Function after Griffiths.* London: London School of Economics.

Gooch S. (1984). No apples for the teacher. *Senior Nurse*, **1**, 8.

Johnson M. (1986). A message for the teacher. *Nursing Times*, **82**: 52, 41–3.

Lelean S. (1973). *Ready for Report Nurse?* London: Royal College of Nursing.

Pyne R. (1987). A professional duty to shout. *Nursing Times*, **83**: 42, 30–1.

Schein E. (1970). *Organisational Psychology*. New Jersey: Prentice Hall.

Sullivan E., Decker P. (1985). *Effective Management in Nursing*. California: Addison-Wesley.

Turnock C. (1987). Task allocation. *Nursing Times*, **83**: 44, 71.

Wrigley S. J., Reynolds M., Whitehead B. (1984). Our teaching isn't dull. *Senior Nurse*, **1**, 12.

14 The ward round

The consultant's ward round is one of the regular rituals of ward life and offers a splendid opportunity to watch what Chapman (1983) describes as the most striking medical ritual of all, the deference ritual. The use of intimidation, mystification and prestige symbols all combine to maintain the status and power of the insiders (consultants) while the outsiders are excluded (everybody else). Berger and Luckman (1975) have written of how the medical profession shrouds itself in the age-old symbols of power and mystery from outlandish costume (the white coat which serves no purpose on the back of a consultant during a ward round) to incomprehensible language (medical jargon). These rituals set the medical profession apart from everybody else and deny entry to all but the chosen few, who in their turn must comply with the ritualistic practices of what at times looks like a cross between the freemasons, a medieval guild and the mafia.

'I expect patients to be weighed daily on my ward, Sister!'
How often have we heard similar comments barked at a nurse in front of the entourage of the ward round. Here the consultant has his captive audience to perform to. Chapman (1983) describes a consultant arriving 2 hours late for his round, demanding that the sister interrupt supervising patient lunches, then ordering her to do four different things at once, all with conflicting priorities. While the sister respectfully tried to do the impossible, he scowled, sighed heavily, tapped his fingers while leaning on the trolley and gazed out of the window. The sister flushed and apologized for being slow in carrying out the impossible tasks demanded of her, complying with the humiliation ritual.

Of course it is not just nursing staff who are treated in this way; medical students and junior doctors receive the same treatment. Is it really necessary to ask a medical student who has an Ambu bag facemask upside down on a patient's face whether the patient's nose is above or below the mouth? Four nurses and another student witnessed this particular consultant's brand of sarcasm and humiliation while the wretched medical student blushed.

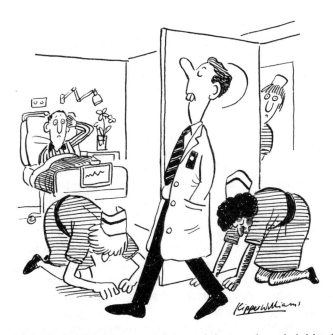

In the field of child abuse it is often said that an abused child is likely to become an abusing parent. Is this also true of the rituals of the medical profession?

Doctors who are rude towards nurses are a sad reality of everyday life. While allowances can be made for doctors who are overworked and, thanks to the bizarre nature of medical shift patterns, have probably had no sleep for the last 36 hours, there are many times when there simply is no excuse. It is part of a ritualistic behaviour pattern that has been learned and reinforced over the years by the passive participation of nurses who allow themselves to be treated in this way. Fortunately there are many doctors who do respect nurses and treat them with the civilities of everyday life, but there are many who do not.

Montgomery (1987) offers an interesting analysis of such situations. She considers verbal abuse to be part of a regular behaviour pattern. Verbal abusers need victims to restore their own feelings of power and control, but they must depersonalize the victim. Thus they see the victim not as Mary Smith, but as a stereotypical nurse, for if she was perceived as a human being this would complicate the situation and make it more difficult. (There are striking parallels here with another male behaviour pattern directed at women, rape.) The victim participates by acquiescing passively to the non-person role by behaving in a stereotypical way, both as a woman and as a nurse.

Acquiescence leads to repetition of the behaviour while confrontation leads to major conflict with management who usually side with the medical staff. Montgomery's analysis offers a way out of the situation, however: humanization is the key. By refusing to acquiesce and behave stereotypically and then humanizing the situation, the nurse can break the ritual humiliation cycle.

Self-control is essential. No matter how hurtful and unjust the criticisms may be, the nurse must maintain an outward appearance of calm despite inner turmoil. It may help to liken this behaviour to the temper tantrum of a 2-year-old and think of this raging tyrant in nappies. All consultants were some mother's son or daughter! The nurse should not argue at this stage as this will be unproductive and only lead to an escalation of hostilities. Rather a straight face, a pause and then, when the storm has abated a little, a firm request to discuss the problem in private away from the audience. If this is refused, the nurse should take the difficult option of following up rather than letting the matter drop and make an appointment to see the consultant later to discuss the issue, via his secretary if necessary.

The aim is to present yourself as a rational human being and a competent caring nurse. As this image is projected and the ward sister becomes more humanized, so it is more difficult for the doctor to engage in verbal abuse. Other staff nurses on the ward may also form targets for abuse. This situation may be alleviated by the subsequent projection of a humanizing image on to all the nursing staff.

This involves a certain amount of assertiveness, what Webb (1987) has described as making one's needs known in a self-confident way and standing firm in defence of one's own and others' rights. Webb is right to advocate nurses taking on a more assertive role and assertiveness training would make a welcome addition to in-service training programmes.

When confronted by an abusive or sarcastic doctor, compliance is as counterproductive as hostile confrontation. An understanding of power rituals and the reasons behind verbal abuse should help the nurse deal with the problem by being assertive and not allowing the offender to depersonalize the situation.

'You are only a nurse, this is my patient!'

A comment such as this conveys the inherent feeling of superiority that characterizes medical thinking. Webster (1988) has described doctors as being typically ethnocentric in their thinking. This term means that a person believes in the inherent superiority of his or her own group and culture and feels contempt for other groups and cultures. (Small wonder some doctors are referred to as 'little Hitlers'!) Webster carried out many interviews with medical students and doctors in her work and concluded that their ethnocentricity leads them to believe that all other health professionals would have been doctors if they could have got into medical school. From this perspective nursing is seen as a lower form of medicine rather than a distinct discipline.

The opposition of the medical profession to many changes in nursing in this country over the last decade stems from their fear of competition. Nursing is seen as a diluted form of medicine which the medical profession must control. How much of the impetus for general management, abolishing as it did the nursing power base, came from behind-the-scenes senior medical sources? It is totally unacceptable that consultants in some areas still sit on sister interview panels. After all, sisters do not appoint consultants.

Although this book is mostly concerned with hospital situations, it is also true to say that there are many seeking to extend medical control over nursing in the community by breaking up the primary health care team concept and replacing it with a system controlled by general practitioners.

This medical domination of nursing is a two-way process for there are many nurses who also see it as the natural order of things. Nursing staff still address the consultant as 'sir' and allow medical staff to take over their office. Some nurses even see nothing wrong with doctors interviewing for nursing posts, a deference that is not reciprocated when consultants are being appointed!

It is impossible to separate the nursing–medical dichotomy without reference to gender. Doctors are usually male and nurses female, with all the implications that has for power and control. Smith (1987) has written that power is the condition of men and the absence of power is the condition of women. She considers it arrogant of doctors to think that nursing has no role other than that defined for it by medicine. It could also be argued that in the past women have had no role other than that defined for them by men and so the two arguments blur into one. The doctor's right to power may well be seen as a myth passed down over the ages (why is the head of a multidisciplinary team always the doctor, asks Smith?) but it is a powerful myth that still has the support of many nurses.

In the previous chapter the issue of the remoteness of role models – sisters – for junior nurses was raised. Junior doctors have very powerful and successful role models close at hand, not so nurses. Even if a sister is in closer contact with her junior staff than the examples considered in the previous chapter, how long is an innovative, bright sister going to remain in that position? Financial necessity or sheer frustration has in the past seen such a sister move on into education, management or outside the National Health Service altogether. If the present regrading exercise is fairly carried out, there is hope that this might not happen so frequently in the future. Regrading may therefore bring about an increase in the number of successful role models for junior nurses in the clinical areas.

However, for many years junior doctors have had successful, powerful role models to emulate, while for female nurses the reverse has been the case. The result has been many nurses and doctors seeing male medical domination as the natural order of things.

Webster's (1988) work concluded that if attitudes are to be changed, social, institutional, interpersonal and personal factors must all be addressed. It is at the interpersonal level that many social and institutional expectations are acted out during professional socialization, therefore this seems an area ripe for action.

Thus female nurses who burst into tears at a male medical tirade are acting out the social stereotype of the female, while the nurse who immediately abandons what she is doing the moment the consultant arrives on the ward to do his round is acting out the institutional stereotype.

A significant, though still small, number of men have come into general hospital nursing in the past 10 years. From personal experience very different attitudes sometimes seem to be displayed by medical staff to male compared to female nurses. Research is needed to describe any such attitude changes with reliability, but sometimes there seems to be more willingness to accept what the male nurse says as an equal (typically from younger doctors) while on other occasions there is more hostility towards a nurse who is male (typically from more senior consultants). If more men stay in clinical nursing it will be interesting to see how medical–nursing relationships develop.

The notion of the patient belonging to the doctor, as in 'my patient', reflects the reality of the power situation between doctors and nurses and also has its origins in legal custom and practice. In the early days of the introduction of the nursing process, many consultants were heard to be very critical of this development as they considered it led to nurses infringing on their areas of responsibility. Not only do consultants talk of 'their' patients but some still talk of 'their nurses' as if they owned the nursing staff on the wards where they have beds.

The traditional 'closed shop' views of some members of the medical profession have more in common with the medieval guild of barber surgeons from which they are descended than with a modern science which has to work closely with other professionals in order to obtain the best results. Teamwork is essential and the best doctors acknowledge this, resulting in a well balanced multidisciplinary approach to care.

Increasingly, the traditional areas of medical supremacy will be challenged by groups such as nurses – it is inherent in the very dynamics of change. A typical example is the challenge presented by community nurses in areas such as the right to prescribe dressings and medications, which has been well argued by Stillwell (1988). As she correctly points out, the theoretical knowledge base of nurses will have to be dramatically improved before such innovative changes can be argued for with any conviction.

'Where is Sister? I want to do my ward round.'

The final question to be addressed in this chapter is whether the sister or her deputy should be involved on the ward round at all. If the ward is running a genuinely multidiscipinary approach, then the full participation of the nursing staff is essential.

However this is not often the case in many hospital specialties, although care of the elderly, mentally handicapped and mentally ill do offer many excellent exceptions. If the ward round is primarily a medical consultation which will decide on new investigations, drug therapy or surgery, what is the point of the nurse being present?

The pressures on a ward sister's time are enormous. Can she justify spending half an hour to an hour pushing a trolley round for the consultant if that is her sole contribution to the round? If the medical staff are interested in what nursing staff have to say so the nurse plays an active part in the round, her presence is justified. If that is not the case, she could more profitably be engaged on nursing care; the ward round is a ritual she can do without. The house officer can notify her of decisions made with regard to medical treatments in so far as they affect nursing care at a later time.

Recommendations for good practice

1. Nursing should be seen as an equal but separate discipline from medicine with mutual respect between both practitioners.

2. Sisters should question whether their presence on a ward round
    benefits the nursing care of patients.

References

Berger P., Luckman T. (1975). *The Social Construction of Reality*. Harmondsworth:
Penguin.
Chapman G. E. (1983). Ritual and rational action in hospitals. *Journal of Advanced
Nursing*, **1**, 13–20.
Montgomery C. (1987). Taming a tyrant. *American Journal of Nursing*, Feb:
234–8.
Smith L. (1987). Doctors rule OK? *Nursing Times*, **83**: 30, 49–51.
Stillwell B. (1988). Should nurses prescribe? *Nursing Times*, **84**: 12, 31–4.
Webb C. (1987). Professionalism revisited. *Nursing Times*, **83**: 35, 39–41.
Webster D. (1988). Medical students and nurses. *Nursing Outlook*, **36**, 130–5.

15 The nursing process

The nursing process was heralded as a major innovation which was going to revolutionize nursing, resulting in a far higher standard of care for patients and more job satisfaction for nurses. It is the method of nursing which must be employed in all teaching areas in order for them to be approved for training by the national boards and it forms the basis for classroom nurse education.

The nursing process is also misunderstood and abused by nurses from one end of the country to the other. In practice it is probably used in something like its intended form in only a small minority of wards. National board inspectors may come and go, care plans are carefully written up as an academic exercise for their visit, but between times, the care given bears little resemblance to the hopes and ideals of those brave enough to try to change British nursing with this concept.

What has gone wrong with this brave new idea? Why has writing care plans become little more than a meaningless ritual? How much substance is there to the criticisms that abound concerning the nursing process? Are these criticisms just another group of myths?

'When I had a bath book at least I knew everybody got a bath.'

The traditional system of organizing nursing care was the task-centred approach with nurses being assigned specific tasks to perform for all patients. Thus two nurses would 'do the back round' and another nurse would 'do the TPR round'. Often a ward book would be kept with a list of tasks to be ticked off by the nurses as they completed their tasks.

The critics of this system point out that it prevents patients being seen as individuals; they are reduced to a collection of tasks. All that nurse A might see of a patient is his or her bottom when it is washed every two hours, whether it needs washing or not. The fragmented nature of this care greatly reduces communication between patient and nurse and leads to psychological and social problems being totally ignored. It must also be said that there was no guarantee that any of the tasks were done. Lelean's work (1973) has already been cited as evidence of this and Chapman (1983) observed students on a 'TPR round' making up temperatures and pulse rates to fill in the charts. Dissatisfaction with the perception that nursing has merely become a series of ritualized tasks might help explain such findings. There is plenty of anecdotal evidence to support Chapman and Lelean's findings.

The task allocation system was very centralized as the nurse in charge for the day decided which patients needed what tasks performed. There was no scope for individual initiative. Decisions about care were seldom based on any rational assessment of the patients' problems, they reflected routine and the opinions of the nurse in charge. The patient's opinion was rarely sought.

It is against this sort of background that the nursing process emerged as a means of rationalizing patient care. The aim was to provide care relevant to the individual patient's needs which acknowledged that the patient was a human being with a mind of his or her own who had to be seen as part of a social setting, and not just a bottom that needed washing every 2 hours. The term *individualized patient care* is in fact a far better term than *nursing process*, for it is an accurate description of what the nurse should be trying to achieve.

'We did have an afternoon session on the nursing process a few years ago, well, sort of . . . .'

On many wards today the nursing process is practised in name only. Nurses have only a vague idea of what it means. Their introduction to this major new concept probably consisted of a 2-hour session on how to fill the forms in at the in-service training department 6 years ago and the delivery of several wheelbarrow-loads of documentation to their ward the following Monday.

The fundamental problem is that the concept was introduced without proper preparation. It is doubtful if many educationalists fully understood what it entailed, and certainly very few nurse managers did. The first step should have been to establish the case for change, before explaining the concept of individualized patient care, its advantages and the various stages in the nursing process. The next stage should have been to involve staff in its implementation by a consultative process including allowing ward staff to design their own care plans.

Logically a trial should have followed with perhaps one or two wards experimenting with the system. A crucial element of such a trial is establishing criteria that demonstrate changes in care received by patients. This lack of an appropriate measuring tool remains a major criticism of much of the work that has been carried out trying to compare the nursing process with traditional nursing. After such trials alterations and improvements could have been made, before introducing the concept into the whole hospital. Again the exact format could be allowed to vary between wards and units as each clinical area is different and will have slightly different requirements in any system of care. Given the authoritarian style that characterizes nurse management (see p. 127), it is not surprising that this consultative approach was not used, as it is more in line with an enlightened democratic style. The system of introduction guaranteed that the nursing process would not be understood by nurses and that it would arouse strongly negative attitudes.

'We don't do the nursing process on lates and at night.'

This frequently heard statement conveys a lack of understanding of what the nursing process involves. It also suggests that the ward does not use the nursing process at all.

To the average nurse the nursing process means patient allocation and care plans. Patient allocation is usually practised on an early shift and involves team nursing. A ward might be split into two or three teams with the result that for that morning 2 or 3 nurses might be responsible for 8–10 patients. Will this guarantee individualized patient care based on a rational assessment of need?

Various writers, such as Turnock (1987), have pointed out that this leads to task-oriented nursing, only on a smaller scale. The back round now involves 8 or 10 patients instead of 30. Tasks are still performed according to the sort of hierarchy examined in the last chapter, with the junior staff doing 'basic' tasks while the third-year student or staff nurse does the complicated dressing. The patient does not receive integrated care.

At lunchtime another team takes over, or no team at all if the ward does not allocate patients to teams in the afternoon and evening. In the first case care is fragmented as two new nurses take over the patient; in the latter case the patient is left with no nurse at all responsible for his or her care.

A nurse may only care for the same patient perhaps two or three times in a week, with the result that the nurse does not get to know the patient and the patient sees a bewildering succession of nurses. Patient allocation carried out in this way fails to meet the need of individualized care and is not the 'nursing process'.

The second element in the average nurse's conception of the nursing process is the care plan; this, more than anything, is the subject of a barrage of nursing criticism. The first problem is that the documentation was rarely designed by the staff who have to use it and the notion that the same form can be used in all the different clinical units of a health authority is laughable. However, autocratic nursing management has ensured that this is the case, leaving staff to struggle with unsuitable documentation.

Even allowing for poor documentation, experience shows that many nurses still do not understand how to devise a care plan. The theory of care-planning is simply not practised. Assessments tend to include much irrelevant information as nurses automatically complete every box on the form. 'Admitting Mr Smith' has become a great ritual. A student nurse confronts the patient with a clipboard and several impressive-looking pieces of paper and proceeds to ask a barrage of questions in order to fill in all the spaces on the form.

Does the nurse then sit down and start to work out patient problems, whether potential or actual, checking out her analysis with the patient to see how he or she feels about possible problems? Of course not. She usually copies out a series of standard statements in tortuous mangled English from another patient's plan without a thought about the patient's individual needs!

Problems are written as nursing problems not those of the patient. The same comment applies to goals. Phrases such as 'to monitor' and 'to prevent' are dotted about the goals column; who will prevent what? Interventions are standardized and vague while the whole plan is usually several days out of date and it is not unusual to find plans untouched by the nurse's pen for weeks and even months.

Using the criterion that a nursing care plan should allow a new nurse to carry out the patient's care for a shift, many care plans are unsatisfactory. Time is frequently wasted asking staff when a patient's dressing was last performed; information such as the frequency of dressing change, materials to be used and the wound appearance at the last dressing change is not recorded. The staff nurse who last did the dressing may be on days off and as there is nothing written in the care plan except an entry 5 days ago along the lines of 'wound, daily dressing', it is not surprising that there is so much discontinuity of care and time wasted.

Care plans have often become a series of standardized entries which have not been amended for days, and which tell the nurse nothing about the care required. Phrases such as 'up and about' and 'push fluids' abound, but they are meaningless when scrutinized carefully. The phrase 'up and about' does not specify how many times the patient should get out of bed in a day, how long at each time, or how far the patient may walk, aided or unaided. 'Push fluids' does not tell the nurse what quantity of fluid is required, or what sorts of fluids are to be encouraged.

The team nursing approach is a major contributory factor to this sort of confusion as no one nurse is responsible for the patient's care. The best analogy is to think of the patient as a basketball and the ward a basketball court. Two teams bounce the ball around, back and forth, while changing their personnel all the time. No one player can tell you much about the ball or where it will go next except that it will end up in one of two baskets eventually. Those two teams are like the teams of nurses on a ward – the baskets are either the mortuary trolley or the hospital exit door.

Individualized patient care (nursing process, if you prefer) is not being effectively practised in many areas. Care plans are often unused which, given the unsatisfactory standards they often reach, is perhaps just as well. The discussion above leads to the following conclusions why this may be:

1. The mode of introduction was authoritarian and inappropriate.
2. The concepts were never fully explained to staff.
3. The focus was on documentation not care. The documentation introduced is often inappropriate.
4. Team nursing means no one nurse is responsible for any patient's care on a 24-hour, day-by-day basis.

Before proceeding to offer some practical suggestions to improve this situation, we need to examine briefly some more popular myths about the nursing process.

'There's too much paperwork. There isn't time for nursing with all that form-filling.'

This reflects the obsession with paperwork and the nursing process, probably stemming from the bureaucratic mentality of many of those responsible for its implementation.

The focus of the nursing process must be the patient, not the paperwork. All the paper does is document what has been done as a record and ensure that a nurse coming on duty knows what is to be done for any one patient in the forthcoming shift – nothing more and nothing less. The nursing process is first and foremost a way of thinking about nursing; it is a rational problem-solving approach.

Supposing you have just had a shower and find that the hairdrier will not work. In everyday life we assess a situation and decide what the problem is (the hairdrier will not work) and decide on a goal (it will work). Then we decide what has to be done in order to achieve that goal (try a new plug) and do it (change the plug). Finally we look to see if it has worked (switch the hairdrier on again). This is all the nursing process consists of. There is nothing high-powered about it and nothing that involves spending hours getting writer's cramp.

If the nurse approaches her or his everyday nursing care with this hairdrier example in mind, she or he will be practising the nursing process. Thus in an area like Accident & Emergency this approach will allow the nurse to practise the nursing process in a situation involving many dozens of patients in a shift, with little or no documentation (Walsh, 1985). The nursing process is merely a logical way of thinking about nursing care.

With regard to the documentation, it should be evaluated critically to see if lengthy assessment forms can be cut down and made relevant to the patient's needs. Patients admitted for day surgery on their ingrowing toenail do not need in-depth assessments taking over half an hour, yet experience shows this may still happen. Because there is a box on the form, nurses feel obliged to fill it in, even though it is irrelevant to patient care and wastes time.

Documenting care actually saves time. It saves the nurse spending 15 minutes trying to find the nurse who did the dressing yesterday and who knows what is to be used, or the nurse in charge to see if a patient can go to the toilet or should use a commode. By speeding up communication in this way, an up-to-date care plan does save time.

Time may also be saved by the use of common core care plans. This approach has been well described on a medical unit by Glasper et al (1987). The authors found that 48–72 hours after admission patients still did not have care plans and on other wards care plans had been abandoned altogether. Common core plans changed this situation completely.

Core care plans are preprinted in advance of admission and drawn up by the staff of a ward considering the various problems commonly faced by most patients on their ward. With care for common problems planned in advance, time is available to concentrate on individual problems. This approach has been described in other areas such as Accident & Emergency by Walsh (1985) and intensive care by Foster (1987). Surgical wards could also benefit from care planning. Individual problems must never be lost sight of, however.

Use of care-planning can improve continuity of care and save time if carried out in a rational manner. Ritualistic filling in of forms however will waste time and be of no benefit to the patient.

'They've proved the nursing process does not work anyway.'
This is a dangerous myth stemming from misreading of the few studies that attempted to compare traditional task-centred care with a team nursing, individualized care-planning approach. Firstly it has to be said that research never proves anything. It suggests or shows things with varying degrees of probability, but there can never be 100% proof of anything. The real world is too complicated for that.

A typical study which has given rise to this myth is that of Berry and Metcalfe (1986) whose results are similar to earlier studies. They investigated the differences found on changing from a task-centred approach to team nursing with care plans in a maternity ward. The results were that the patients found no difference, although the midwives preferred the new system as it gave them more job satisfaction. This has been a typical finding of many such studies.

The researchers point out that there is a big difference between a midwifery ward and a general hospital ward as the mothers are much more involved in their own care and the care of their babies than are patients on a typical ward. They went on to cast doubt upon how effectively the ward staff had really changed their practice (a comment that may be made about other such studies) and made their most telling point when discussing the sensitivity of their measuring tool.

Most studies have relied on a patient questionnaire with very broad questions about general satisfaction with care. Is such a tool sensitive enough to measure improvements in care? The researchers think not and urge the development of more specific and sensitive ways of measuring the standard of care. After all, patient temperature is measured with a thermometer rather than the palm of the hand placed on the patient's brow, and if a recipe calls for 100 g of flour, it is measured with kitchen scales rather than a weighbridge.

The methods used to evaluate the effect of the nursing process on patients in most studies to date are acknowledged by researchers to have been inadequate and the validity of the studies has been open to serious question.

One study has used different tools and come up with different answers. Miller (1985) measured length of stay in hospital and patient dependency. This study showed a reduction in both after the implementation of the nursing process. Individualizing patient care led to less dependent patients who could be discharged earlier. The statement that the nursing process has been proved not to work is therefore a myth.

Task-centred nursing has been rejected and the notion of individualized care using patient-centred planning (the nursing process) advocated. There are serious doubts about how effectively team nursing can deliver individualized patient care. The solution to this problem is the notion of primary nursing which has been well described by Wright (1987) and MacGuire (1988) in two different settings. In brief, primary nursing involves one nurse having overall responsibility for a patient's care whether the nurse is on duty or not. That nurse assesses the patient and plans care accordingly. When she or he is not on duty other nurses follow the care plan, updating it as needed.

One nurse is thus responsible for 24 hours. This is individualized nursing care compared to the team nursing situation where nobody is responsible, not even the team leader, for more than a few hours at a time. Correct documentation thus becomes essential if a care plan is to be effective. If a nurse knows that a patient and his or her care plan is that nurse's professional responsibility throughout a patient's stay in hospital, there should be a dramatic improvement in care-planning. Continuity of care is more likely to be achieved in this way.

In this chapter we have seen that unfortunately the nursing process has led to much ritualistic filling in of forms and has generated a substantial amount of mythology. Autocratic management and poor teaching got the nursing process off to the worst possible start and have contributed to the fact that in many areas care remains task-centred, disjointed and lacking in individuality.

Recommendations for good practice

1. The term *nursing process* should be abandoned and replaced by *individualized patient care*, a more accurate description.
2. A major re-education campaign is needed to improve nurses' care-planning ability.
3. Wards should be encouraged to adopt their own documentation, with the development of core care plans if appropriate.
4. Primary nursing should become the method of delivering individualized patient care, replacing team nursing.
5. Appropriate measuring tools should be devised to monitor the quality of nursing care at present and in the aftermath of such a change.

References

Berry A. J., Metcalfe C. L. (1986). Paradigms and practices, the organisation of the delivery of nursing care. *Journal of Advanced Nursing*, **11'**, 589–97.

Chapman G. E. (1983). Ritual and rational action in hospitals. *Journal of Advanced Nursing*, **1**, 13–20.

Foster D. (1987). The development of care plans for the critically ill patient. *Nursing*, **31**, 571–3.

Glasper A., Stonehouse J., Martin L. (1987). Core care plans. *Nursing Times*, **83**: 10, 55–7.

Lelean S. (1973). *Ready for Report Nurse?* London: Royal College of Nursing.

MacGuire J. (1988). I'm your nurse. *Nursing Times*, **84**: 30, 32–6.

Miller A. (1985). Nurse patient dependency; is it iatrogenic? *Journal of Advanced Nursing*, **10**, 1.

Turnock C. (1987). Task allocation. *Nursing Times*, **83**: 44, 71.

Walsh M. (1985). A&E nursing: A New Approach. Oxford: Heinemann.

Wright S. (1987). Patient centred practice. *Nursing Times*, **83**: 38, 24–7.

16 Rituals and the challenge of research

This book has described nursing care as it is in the real world, rather than as it ought to be, which is the usual textbook approach. We have seen that mythology abounds and many aspects of nursing care are ritualistic and demonstrably of no value, if not positively harmful to patients.

In this final chapter the question must be addressed of why this is so. Nursing before 1970 did not possess any significant research base and could not be said to have a body of knowledge unique to itself. However, the last 20 years has seen a steady expansion in nursing research which has shown many nursing practices to be useless, yet the rituals persist. This indicates that a fundamental problem exists in translating the findings of research into British nursing practice.

It is worth looking at how receptive American nurses are to research findings. A study by Luckenbill-Brett (1987) investigated the research awareness of 216 practising registered nurses in hospitals of all sizes in the USA. She focused on 14 different research findings covering topics from IVI site changes to mutual goal-settings and her results are summarized in Table 4.

Luckenbill-Brett expresses cautious optimism about these results as they do appear to show that there is diffusion of research findings to practising nurses with a limited amount of uptake. The fact that on average 70% of nurses were aware of findings but only 28% said they always implemented them is little cause for rejoicing, however. It would be interesting to undertake a replication of this study on UK nurses to see how they compare with their American colleagues.

Table 4 Awareness of 216 registered nurses of research findings

State of awareness	Mean % for 14 findings
Aware of research findings	70
Persuaded of the value of findings	58
Sometimes implement finding	33
Always implement finding	28

From Luckenbill-Brett (1987).

Is it realistic to expect a single nurse to read a piece of research and then introduce the appropriate changes in to her or his practice? The answer is probably not, as she or he is greeted with comments like: 'Sister likes it done this way' or 'We've always done it that way'. Even if the individual nurse is prepared to brave the slings and arrows of outraged tradition and ritual, she or he will find attempts at change undermined by the other staff on the ward the moment she or he goes off duty. The inertia of nursing is such that a ward always tends to revert to old practices.

If the nurse is to implement change she or he must be aware of the difficulties involved in changing attitudes and beliefs. Claxton (1987) has described beliefs as fixed assumptions people have about the way things are or at least the way they ought to be. Such a belief involves a personal commitment to something being a certain way. It is this personal commitment to beliefs that leads to a resistance to change because if change is threatened, the person tends to resist in order to preserve the view that this is the way things should be. Alternatively he or she may ignore the change altogether, carrying on as if nothing had happened.

If we look at changes in wound-dressing methods or how nursing care should be organized, we can see that we are up against a set of beliefs that experienced nurses hold about the correct lotions and materials which should be used or the benefits of task allocation to get the work done. Nurses tend to hold personal commitments to these beliefs and so resist change, as they see change threatening their very self.

If the history of nursing were different, nursing practice might be based on something more substantial than beliefs and this problem would not exist. Nursing prior to the 1970s unfortunately had little research tradition. In addition it had no sense of a body of professional knowledge unique to nursing; it was devoid of theory except the notion of subservience to medicine. Thus nursing care was not based on nursing fact but rather on what doctors thought nurses ought to know and on an oral tradition of beliefs passed from sister to student. Beliefs therefore became ingrained into the fabric of nursing and mistaken for facts.

The work of researchers in the last 20 years has been frustrated in many areas because their findings are challenging beliefs and, as we have seen above, people have a personal commitment that leads them to ignore facts which challenge their beliefs. The perception that research nurses are remote from clinical practice and in some way academic or 'high brow' has made it easier for clinical staff to ignore research findings. They can rationalize their way out of the dilemma by statements such as: 'That's all very well in theory, but you just don't appreciate what it's like in the real world of my ward'.

Research in nursing will be greatly helped by bringing the researchers and clinicians closer together. It will also be aided by research nurses writing up their findings in language that is accessible to all, rather than resorting to difficult jargon which few nurse clinicians can understand.

The tradition of subservience in nursing represents a further stumbling block to change. As an agent of change the nurse will probably have to deal with senior nurses, doctors and managers. Subservience is of little value here. What is needed is assertiveness, and this is sadly lacking, not only because of the subservient tradition of nursing, but also because as most nurses are women, they have been socially conditioned out of any assertive tendencies they may have.

We would urge future curriculum designers to build assertiveness training into their educational programmes for students, and to recognize assertiveness as an essential skill for any nurse in just the same way as the ability to read or perform mathematical calculations. In the meanwhile, nurses should be lobbying their in-service training units to lay on assertiveness workshops. We believe such skills are essential to remove the dead hand of tradition in nursing and for clinicians to grow into people with the strength to implement change.

This analysis of resistance to change in nursing suggests some useful ways forward. Firstly we must ensure that nursing practice in the future is not based purely upon beliefs, but rather is a rational, fact-based discipline, therefore more susceptible to change in the face of research findings and new ideas. Nursing will always need a fundamental belief system about the very nature of nursing – a broad philosophy of care – but that should not be confused with beliefs about the best way to dress a wound or prepare a patient for theatre.

Nursing may consider its fundamental belief system or philosophy of care through the concept of nursing models. Writers such as Henderson, Roy and Orem have all proposed theoretical constructs or models of what nursing is. They have attempted to identify a body of knowledge unique to nursing and underpinned it with a basic philosophy of care. Orem, for example, bases her model on the notion that nursing is aimed at assisting patients and their families to achieve self-care, while Roy suggests nursing should be concerned with helping patients to adapt to stressors to achieve health. These stressors may be physical, psychological and social in origin.

Beliefs about nursing come into play at this philosophical level for they also include the individual nurse's belief system about what is right and wrong. Nurses must not be judgemental about patients and they must remember that patients will probably have different belief systems from their own. These differences, seeing things from the patient's point of view, are an essential ingredient of good nursing care. However we must not confuse beliefs about the best way to heal a pressure sore with the demonstrated facts and it is the incorporation of individual, idiosyncratic beliefs into nursing care at this level that is responsible for many of the problems identified in this book.

If nurses wish to try and change practice today, they must learn the lessons that psychology can teach us about changing attitudes and beliefs. While it is difficult to change attitudes, it is also possible, and the key to unlocking the door of change is known as cognitive dissonance theory. This theory suggests that if we have an attitude that something is wrong or will not work, but we then operate with that something for a while and the experience that follows shows that it does work, we have a problem in reconciling our knowledge with our belief. This reconciliation can often be shown to lead to a change in attitude − a change that would not have occurred by simple attempts at persuasion.

A good example of this theory at work on a grand scale was the racial integration of education in the USA in the 1960s. Opponents argued that white children did not know enough about blacks to share the same school. There would have to be a massive education programme to teach whites about blacks before schools could be integrated or else the result would be total disruption of the education system brought about by inter-racial violence. Others of course said whites and blacks could never be integrated at all. Cognitive dissonance theory (Hilgard et al 1987) predicted that is schools were integrated, whites would have to reconcile their attitudes to blacks with their knowledge gained at first hand by sharing the same classroom (and vice versa), the result being that the two races would get along in integrated schools.

Experience has shown that cognitive dissonance worked. While there remain significant racial tensions and disharmony in American society, they are far less pronounced than the opponents of integration predicted.

If this approach is to be applied to nursing it suggests that change is closely bound up with doing rather than just talking. Theory suggests that attitudes to dressings might best be changed by introducing a new technique and inviting nurses to see how it works. They must then reconcile the demonstrable improvement with their belief that there will be no improvement.

There is an immediate pitfall to be avoided; that is the traditional autocratic approach of some elements of nurse management which might lead to a new procedure being introduced by dictate. There should of course be consultation and explanation, the point should be made that this is only a trial for a limited period and the change should be introduced in such a way as to be as non-threatening as possible to the nursing staff.

A skilful way of presenting change is for the manager to try and guide a group to their own solutions to problems. Thus one member of the group might be invited to look at an aspect of care firstly to identify that there is a problem, since without recognition of the need for change, change will never occur. Again the manager may then try and use other group members to come up with solutions which can then be tried in practice, hoping for the cognitive dissonance effect to occur. In this context, the term *manager* could mean a ward sister or clinical nurse specialist.

The process of change requires everyone to accept the possibility of making errors during the transitional period. Who learnt to drive without making a few errors? This is of course a threat to a person's self-esteem and may be so severe that it inhibits him or her from attempting change. The nurse therefore needs to feel able to make the inevitable mistakes that will occur in trying a new technique if change is to be encouraged. The nurse will also tend to be aware of being different during a change. This too can cause difficulties as people do not like being different, they prefer to conform in order to gain acceptance. These points should guide how nursing staff attempt to implement change during the trial period.

If a nurse is to change practice she or he must recognize that she or he is seeking to challenge another nurse's beliefs. This entails challenging something to which the nurse has a personal commitment. By making that nurse change you are demanding that she or he pays the price of being different and of possible failure with the new technique. Cognitive dissonance theory shows a way forward to help change attitudes and beliefs, but this makes heavy demands which require a careful strategy, involving support to help the nurse cope with doing something different and possibly failing to get it right at first.

A major study of the problems of introducing research findings was carried out by Hunt (1987) who confirmed the difficulties involved in change. Hunt studied practices relating to preoperative fasting and mouth care and concluded that the processes necessary to implement change in the light of research were beyond the capacity of any one nurse. The inertia of the system is just too great. There are too many bureaucratic, political, organizational and social factors for any one nurse to tackle. This makes rather depressing reading, so now for some good news. Hunt was able to implement rational change, but only after involving nurse teachers, ward sisters and managers in teams working on identifying the problems, the relevant research literature and the necessary changes in existing practice. With such an enormous expenditure of effort, rational changes became possible, hence Hunt's final conclusion that as much effort needs to be put into the implementation of changes as into the generation of new knowledge.

Confirmation of the value of this team approach comes from Alexander and Orton (1988) who describe a study involving the King's Fund. With the support of this organization, triads were set up consisting of a ward sister, her immediate manager and the teacher with responsibility for her ward. Researchers working with 36 such triads over several years were able to effect research-based change.

The conclusions that may be drawn from these studies are that the nurse who tries to go it alone will be beaten by the system. To bring about rational change in nursing practice requires a major commitment from education and management, as well as clinical staff. There must be recognition of the psychological factors involved in changing beliefs and attitudes. Finally the support of outside agencies is crucial. While there is only one King's Fund, there are over 20 university and polytechnic-based departments of nursing with research expertise available for hospital staff to approach. As much effort as went into the original research is needed if the findings of the work are ever to make their way into nursing practice.

In this book we have shown that while there is a great deal wrong with nursing in some areas, there are also centres of excellence where practice is rational rather than ritualistic. If the hopes and aspirations of Project 2000 are ever to become reality, nursing must abandon ritual and myth and progress to a rational research-based footing. Until such a step is taken it is hard to justify the title of *profession* for nursing. It is better considered a caring *craft*.

References

Alexander M., Orton H. (1988). Research in action. *Nursing Times*, **4**: 8, 38–41.
Clayton G. (1987). Beliefs and behaviour: why is it so hard to change? *Nursing*, **3**, 670–3.

Hunt M. (1987). The process of translating research findings into nursing practice. *Journal of Advanced Nursing*, **2**, 101–10.

Hillgard E., Atkinson R. L., Atkinson C. (1987). *Introduction to Psychology*. New York: Harcourt Brace Jovanovitch Co.

Luckenbill-Brett J. (1987). Use of nursing practice research findings. *Nursing Research*, **36**, 344–9.

Vaughan B., Pearson A. (1986). In *Nursing Models for Practice*. Oxford: Heinemann.

Index

failure in practice, 85–6
mini-round, 85, 86
recommendations for good
practice, 90

Egg white/oxygen, 77, 78
Elderly people, care of, 92–9
myths:
confusion/dementia, 99–100
discharge following, 96–8
health decline, 95–6
incontinence, 93–5
mental ability decline, 92–3
sex, 93
Elderly people, care of,
recommendations for good
practice, 99
Electric clippers, 7
Endotoxin, 28
Endotracheal intubation, 3
Erythema, 66
Erythromycin, 18
European Community, 128
Eusol, 17, 27–8, 31, 78

Femoral temperature taking, 53
Fibroblast, 28
Fibrous products, 31
Flamazine, 31
Fluid balance, chart, 66–8
recommendations for good
practice, 68
Foams, 31
Forceps, disposable plastic, 17
Fucidin tulle, 29

Gauze, 27, 31, 113
unused CSSD packs from, 19
Gauze dressing, 29, 30
Gellperm, 31
Gentian violet, 78
Geriatric ward, 93
Giving set, 24
Glasgow coma scale, 62

Glycerin thymol mouthwash tablets,
113
Graduate nurse, 128–9
Granuflex, 31, 32
Graph, observations, 62
Griffiths report, nursing
management, 87, 126

Haemodynamic condition, unstable,
54
Half-life, 4
Hand-wash, 16
Henderson nursing model, 152
Hepatitis, 113
Hibisol, 17
Hierarchy, nursing within, *see under*
Nursing
Hockey, Lisbeth, 9
Holistic patient-centred care, 84
Hospice movement, 100
Hydrocolloid, 31
Hydrogel, 31
Hydrogen peroxide, 113
Hypochlorite dressings, renal failure
after, 28
Hypochlorite solutions, 17, 27, 28,
33, 81
Hypotension, 60
Hypothermia, 50
Hypovalaemic shock, 60

Imagery, 46
Incontinence, 68–9, 93–5
Individualized patient care, 112, 120,
132, *see also* Nursing process;
Patient-centred care
definition, 142
ineffective practice, 145
practised 24 hours, 116
task-centre care compared, 147
Infection, prevention, 15–25
Inflammatory response, 50
In-service training programme, 59,
80